EAT PRETTY EVERY DAY

365 DAILY INSPIRATIONS

*for nourishing beauty,
inside and out*

Jolene Hart, CHC, AADP

CHRONICLE BOOKS
SAN FRANCISCO

Library of Congress Cataloging-in-Publication Data

Names: Hart, Jolene, author.
Title: Eat pretty every day : 365 daily inspirations for nourishing beauty,
    inside and out / Jolene Hart.
Description: San Francisco : Chronicle Books, [2016] | Includes index.
Identifiers: LCCN 2016021194 | ISBN 9781452151625 (paperback)
Subjects: LCSH: Nutrition. | Beauty, Personal. | Functional foods. | BISAC:
    HEALTH & FITNESS / Beauty & Grooming. | HEALTH & FITNESS / Nutrition.
Classification: LCC RA784 .H3692 2016 | DDC 613.2—dc23 LC record available at https://
lccn.loc.gov/2016021194

Manufactured in China

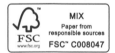

Design by Sydney Goldstein
Illustrations by Vikki Chu
Typesetting by Frank Brayton

10 9 8 7 6

Chronicle Books LLC
680 Second Street
San Francisco, California 94107
www.chroniclebooks.com

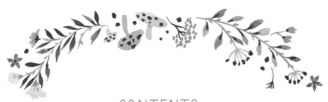

CONTENTS

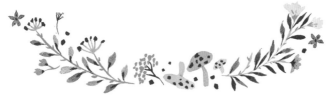

INSPIRATION FOR DAYS

One moment of inspiration can turn your day around. And one moment of inspiration every day of the year can transform your mindset, your routine, and, I deeply believe, the way you look and feel.

The pages of daily inspiration in this book help you create a solid foundation upon which to live your healthy, beautiful, precious life. Some of the entries build upon familiar ideas; they serve as reminders of time-tested ways to nourish health and happiness. Others may be new, and even a bit odd at first; these aim to push your limits and expand your repertoire of habits that support you, every day. You're likely to find some ideas to be surprising, some challenging, and still others effortless— a perfect fit for you. Collectively and over time, reading and acting on these inspirations can restore harmony to your body, heighten the pleasure you get from your relationship with food, raise your consciousness about the transformative power of self-love, shift your thinking, and inspire you to build a lifestyle of beauty that's unique to you and your needs. With every page, and everything you do, you'll be working to transform your beauty, inside and out.

My first book, *Eat Pretty*, introduced the direct ties between food, self-care, and beauty. In this book, *Eat Pretty Every Day*, my goal was to put those powerful connections and the ideas behind them into practice, helping you, the reader, create your own lifestyle of beauty. Season by season and day by day, I want you to feel prepared and motivated to apply beauty nutrition, self-care, and healthy vanity to your routine, with action-oriented goals, recipes, DIY tips, science-backed beauty facts, words of guidance, and essential beauty foods to add to your diet—all of which will help you build a rich and pleasure-packed life that supports you in looking and feeling gorgeous. These pages hold ideas for well-being that I've incorporated into my own lifestyle, foods I stock in my kitchen, and habits I follow consistently to stay on track.

I continue to hear from women around the world that the concepts of beauty nutrition—that is, the foods and nutrients that directly support and enhance our beauty by defending, repairing, and strengthening it—and healthy vanity, or our innate desire to look and feel beautiful, are so relevant in their lives. Those principles certainly resonate in my own life. As a beauty writer at a major fashion magazine, giving beauty advice was my job, but my skin issues and relationship with food left me far from looking and feeling my best, even with access to a staggering array of top beauty products, services, and experts. After looking everywhere *but* inside my own body for answers, I finally found that healing the beauty issues that had plagued me for almost a decade and restoring my belief in my own beauty started, simply enough, with my daily meals—how I approached them as well as what I ate. Employing tools that are neither exclusive nor expensive, I watched my skin transform from painfully blemished, irritated, and inflamed to calm, clear, and healthy. At the same time, I ended my battle with the scale, experienced a surge in energy and positivity that I had struggled for, and felt more true to myself and my body than I had in years. Over time, I've seen and heard firsthand that so many other women have experienced transformations just like mine when they make nutrition a central part of their beauty routines.

More and more, we are learning just how dramatically our mindset creates our reality. When it comes to beauty, the link between mind and matter is incredibly powerful. Yes, you are what you eat—but you are also what you *believe* you are. In light of this, in this book you'll find a deepened focus on self-love and mindfulness and the connection of those factors to beauty. A core belief of the Eat Pretty philosophy is that food isn't your enemy—on the contrary, it can be your greatest tool for beauty. And, like bringing knowledge and intention to your food choices, practicing mindfulness can be a source of great strength, positivity, and beauty in your life. Presenting a year of beauty mapped out before you, day by day, this book is a course in self-discovery that will help you look and feel your most beautiful. This year, do one thing every day that makes you glow.

In beauty and health,

Jolene

HOW TO USE THIS BOOK

Turn to the season you are currently enjoying in your spot on the globe, be it spring, summer, autumn, or winter, and start reading at Day 1. Over the course of more than ninety days, you'll encounter an array of foods, habits, and mindsets—either new to you or renewed—plus instructions and counsel on how to use them to help you nourish optimal beauty and health during that season. If the current season is just a few weeks from its close, then you may want to look ahead to prepare your body and mind for the upcoming shift to the next season, then begin reading from Day 1 when that season arrives. If you're just a few weeks into a new season, then catch up on what you missed until you're up to date and then read on, one entry each day as designed. If you skip a few days, just pick up where you left off. And if you feel motivated to read ahead, go for it!

As the days pass and you absorb the guidance and explore the many benefits offered in these pages, listen carefully to your body to discover what truly makes you look and feel your best. What foods and habits help you feel radiant? Which ideas get you excited, and fit naturally with your personality and lifestyle? I hope you'll trust your inherent knowledge of your body's own needs, but approach each new day with an open mind, letting these daily inspirations lead you to discoveries and breakthroughs on your own journey to your most beautiful self.

YOUR YEAR-ROUND BEAUTY JOURNEY

Open a magazine or turn on the television, and you're bound to see advertisements for lipstick, anti-aging cream, and other magic elixirs that promise youthfulness, beauty, and radiance. But if you're reading this book, chances are you've discovered that these "quick fixes"—while they can certainly serve as fun indulgences—don't build the long-term beauty that you're seeking. What *does* build beauty is a balance of daily diet and lifestyle choices and attentiveness to your mindset, outlook, and self-perception. Real, beautiful results come from ordinary, everyday actions that have the power to affect a dramatic overall change in the way you look and feel. Life, as no doubt you've heard before, is the journey more than the destination. Well, so is beauty. You make certain decisions along the path of your journey and, insignificant as they seem right then and there, they may end up being incredibly impactful for the beauty you aim to see and feel tomorrow, and into the future. Those little habits can become the foundation of your lifestyle, your mindset, and even your identity.

This book is full of inspiration for making our daily moments of nourishment and self-care into something larger and lasting and beautiful, physically and mentally. Too often, our beauty routine is driven by a response to the things we see in the mirror: a new crop of blemishes, lackluster hair, fine lines, or extra pounds. It's not until we notice an issue that we start to freak out—and actually try to *do* something about it. Whether or not you are feeling the need for a tune-up or a change, the ideas in this book will shift not only how you look and feel in the short term, but the way you will age if you make them into habits. I challenge you to start investing in your beauty and body today, whether you're sixteen or sixty. It'll bring you confidence and great pleasure (and likely save you money on health and beauty costs in the years ahead!). As you page through the daily entries in this book, resolve to start taking the best care of your beauty at this moment, whatever season you may be in, even with one very simple new action that you take *right now*.

➤➤ THE EAT PRETTY ESSENTIALS ◄◄

As you begin to build your lifestyle of beauty this year—and anytime you need to reset your inner beauty compass—ask yourself the following essential questions. They will bring you to the heart of the Eat Pretty philosophy and guide you along your journey.

What's feeding your beauty?

"Beauty nutrition" refers to the power of your food to transform the way you look and feel. It's the foundation of the Eat Pretty approach to beauty. The food you eat doesn't just give you energy to go, go, go—it supports your body's beautifying processes, turns on and shuts off genes that influence the way your body performs, and tells your body whether to slow or speed up the aging process. What's more, your food breaks down into molecular building blocks that *become* your body, so it follows that choosing the best food produces your most radiant self. There are so many exciting ways to boost the quality and quantity of the nutritional tools you give your body to defend, repair, detox, and feel its best, and you'll find them filling nearly every page of this book!

What's keeping you from your best self?

Is a mindset or belief holding you back? A negative job or relationship? Or could your diet even play a role, by working against your best efforts to feel beautiful? Some foods out there do just that. I call them the Beauty Betrayers: the foods that don't do any favors for your skin, your body, and your overall beauty. They may taste wonderful in the moment, but long-term, they're making it harder for you to get the glow you're seeking. And while they are impossible to avoid *all* the time, limiting your intake of the following offenders will boost your beauty in big ways.

BEAUTY BETRAYERS

ALCOHOL is a source of simple sugars that stresses the liver (a key organ for radiant skin) and speeds up the aging process.

CAFFEINE increases the stress hormone cortisol, which contributes to wrinkling and belly fat and inhibits the natural production of serotonin, an important happiness booster. Caffeine also alters blood sugar, impedes the absorption of several key beauty minerals, places an additional burden on the body's adrenal glands and liver, and can disrupt beauty sleep, even twelve hours after consumption.

CANNED FOODS WITH BPA (BISPHENOL A) pass an endocrine-disrupting chemical into your system that can throw off the body's delicate hormonal balance.

DAIRY, both organic and conventional, is a common food intolerance that can produce digestive issues. Conventional dairy in particular contains antibiotics and hormones that may affect the body's hormonal balance as well as insulin levels, contributing to breakouts.

FRIED FOODS are a source of heated oils and trans fats that are inflammatory and high in aging free radicals that cause cellular damage.

GLUTEN is a common food sensitivity that can negatively impact digestion and increase levels of inflammation, contributing to breakouts, weight gain, and an advanced rate of aging.

GRILLED AND OVERCOOKED FOODS are known to contain high levels of advanced glycation end products (AGEs), which speed up visible signs of aging such as wrinkles, age spots, and sagging skin, as well as increase inflammation and weight gain.

MEATS (CONVENTIONAL) often contain antibiotics, hormones (both added and natural), and an abundance of omega-6 fats that raise levels of inflammation. Choose organic, grass-fed meats in small amounts, or substitute beautifying protein sources like wild salmon, sardines, and pastured eggs that are high in anti-inflammatory omega-3s and other beauty nutrients, as well as plant-based proteins like quinoa, hemp seeds, and lentils, which offer healthy fats, fiber, and an array of nutrients.

PESTICIDE-SPRAYED PRODUCE is a major source of pesticide residue that increases free radicals in the body, affects hormonal balance, and contributes to a greater toxic burden in the body. (See "A Note on Organic Foods," ahead.)

PROCESSED FOODS are low in beauty nutrition and high in inflammatory compounds like preservatives, chemical additives, synthetic dyes, added flavors, and sugar. They often rank high on the glycemic index and can be a major factor in breakouts and advanced aging.

SODA is sugar-packed and highly acidic in the body. Diet versions can slow metabolism, disrupt healthy gut bacteria, and throw off blood sugar balance.

SUGAR, in its many forms but especially the processed and refined varieties, directly contributes to wrinkles, age spots, blemishes, lackluster skin, cellulite, and weight gain. It steals nutrients and hydration from your skin, suppresses the immune system, increases inflammation, negatively impacts blood sugar balance, and curbs the production of anti-aging hormones in the body.

How does your body receive food?

This question can be broken into two parts: 1) What are your mood, mindset, and environment like when you sit down to eat? And 2) Is your body physically at its best to break down and assimilate the nutrients in your meals? Even the most nourishing meal of healthy, organic ingredients can work against your body if it's not digested well, preventing it from utilizing the beautifying nutrients in your food. Everything from stress, poor diet, and rushed and distracted eating to pesticides and food allergies can negatively impact the beneficial bacteria in your body that is so critical for immunity, mood, resilience to stress, and lifelong beauty and health. One of our goals throughout this year is to strengthen your digestive health and build positive rituals into your mealtime so you'll notice a visible beauty boost.

What motivates you?

One key factor that should drive your creation of a beautifying lifestyle is what I call healthy vanity. Healthy vanity is your desire to look and feel your best, and to show that best self to the world—defining "best self" however you choose! We all possess healthy vanity to some degree. Tap into that force within yourself, and use it for motivation not only to apply to the challenges and the knowledge in this book, but to create a lifestyle that makes you feel your best—and keep it going year after year. You deserve to look and feel like your best self every day, so don't settle until you find the foods, habits, and thoughts that get you there.

What does your daily routine look like?

Look at an average day in your life, and break it down into the individual parts that make up the whole of your health, happiness, and beauty. If there are parts that don't suit you any longer, habits that need refreshing, or situations that need to change, act on them this year. Feeling like you have a daily routine that supports your best self provides unmatched energy for your personal beauty journey.

Consider what a year in your life looks like, month by month and season by season. The needs of your beauty and body shift throughout the seasons and your life, in a cyclical way, which is why you'll find the ideas in this book organized to reflect the seasons of the year. Each season of the year offers unique foods with benefits that closely target the most prominent beauty needs of that time, which is why seasonal eating is a key element to the Eat Pretty philosophy. Get in touch with the natural cycles around you, nuanced according to your environment, age, and even your personality, and use the seasonal cycles to embrace new foods, welcome changes, and inspire new goals.

A NOTE ON ORGANIC FOODS

In a perfect world, organic produce would be free, or at least consistently affordable, for every individual. Imagine never having to weigh the cost of organic blueberries against the pesticide exposure you may receive from conventional berries, or against this week's grocery budget. While buying organic is a very worthy investment, not everyone has the means or the access to purchase all organic all the time. I encourage you to purchase organic versions of as much of your food as possible. However, in this book I've adopted some middle ground: I specify organic versions of all produce that appears on the list of most pesticide-sprayed produce, like peppers and grapes. When you see "organic" specified in a recipe, you'll know that buying the organic version of this food is a top-priority investment in your beauty and health.

While I urge you to reflect on these questions, know that there's no such thing as a perfect answer or a secret beauty formula. There are no hard-and-fast rules when so much of our beauty relies on our individual bodies and feelings. This book starts you on a path, and gives you ideas when you run dry or you're in need of motivation. Just the act of flipping through it is a little bit of self-love; these pages hold a reservoir of inspiration and ideas that you can turn to daily to keep up your momentum, and cull together a year of moments that I hope will reinforce your beautiful life, as it goes on and on.

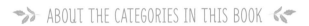

ABOUT THE CATEGORIES IN THIS BOOK

The 365 entries filling the pages ahead fall into nine different categories. Each category represents a distinct aspect of our lives that is essential to nourishing our beauty, inside and out. From recipes and scientific studies to thought-provoking mantras and action-oriented to-dos, there's something unique in each entry to help you build beauty into every one of your days.

Mealtime Mantras

Pausing for a moment of mindfulness before taking the first bite of your meal helps you to be both present and grateful, and to fully taste each mouthwatering, beautifying bite. A mealtime mantra—a positive affirmation you call to mind before eating, or anytime during the day when your outlook needs a lift—creates an opportunity for that thoughtful, reflective moment. The way you receive your meals, including your environment and emotional state, impacts the beauty you derive from it. Shifting your mind away from your to-do list, your inbox, or the television helps you to see the abundance and beauty offered to you on your plate.

Intentions of the Week

Setting intentions and working toward them is an essential aspect of any major transformation. I've broken down some of the core tenets of *Eat Pretty* and turned them into weekly aspirations that you can use to build your lifestyle of beauty, week by week, over the course of the year. Keep in mind that these entries present goals to strive for, which are meant to encourage you to try new things or shake off old habits and mindsets that could be holding you back. They won't all be easy, but they're sure to pass on significant beauty benefits just in the attempt, and give big results if you complete them.

Beauty Food Profiles

There is a world of beautifying food out there, and the best way to build your beauty diet is to focus on the foods that nourish and deepen your glow, rather than out of temptation or habit, dwelling on foods that undermine your glow. You'll find in-depth looks at dozens of new beauty foods in the pages ahead, to complement the list of nearly one hundred beauty foods found in *Eat Pretty*.

Kitchen Inspirations

You're beginning to recognize which foods nourish your body and beauty, but it's not always easy or obvious how to turn them into regular staples in your diet. Entries in this category offer creative ways to incorporate the most beautifying foods into your meals, rethink old cooking and eating habits, and transform the time you spend in the kitchen. Whether you're a total beginner or a devoted cook, you're guaranteed to pick up some new ideas in these entries. And with the right inspiration, the real goal—getting you into the kitchen to prepare nourishing foods—becomes effortless.

Time for Self-Love

Pampering should be easy, right? Who can't make time for some self-love, be it in the form of a healthy meal, a spa moment, or some downtime with a favorite hobby? But believe it or not—although I'm guessing you've experienced this, too—simply finding ways to love and care for themselves is often the task that my clients struggle with the most. Scientific research around mindfulness and self-love is exploding, with one recent study finding that practicing the two correlates to increased resilience (a quality strongly tied to youthfulness) and even better sleep (perhaps the most underappreciated part of our daily beauty routine). This is your year to get serious about self-love, and see the results in the mirror.

Pretty Pairings

Some foods complement each other not only in taste, but also in their beauty-boosting powers. Eating them together enhances their beauty benefits by enabling you to process or absorb more of their nutrients, or creating additional benefits for your body like making you feel more satiated, or reducing the blood sugar spike that results. These beauty food combinations (some of my very favorites) will please your palate and create nutritional nirvana at the same time.

Eat Pretty Recipes

If I could hang out with you in your kitchen, the recipes I included in this book are the beauty-boosting meals that we'd make together. They offer the qualities that you want in the foods on an Eat Pretty plate: colorful, rich in nutrients, anti-inflammatory, fresh, and seasonal. There's a little something for every taste: from sweets to savories and snacks to dinner. Sample a range of these recipes and see if they're meals that *your* body loves.

Beauty Science

The science of beauty—including findings not just on nutrition but also the interplay of sleep, stress, human connection, and enjoyment of nature, among other themes—is an area of incredibly fascinating exploration. These entries detail some of the most exciting new discoveries and ongoing research that inform the way we look and feel each day, and the way we age. Fundamentally, many of the guidelines around your beauty diet and your self-care come from your own understanding of your body, but I think you may find that scientific research backs up many of your personal findings as well!

Living Your Best Life

These activity-inspired entries encourage you to create a life that makes you look and feel your best every day. You might learn how to streamline meal prep, detox your deodorant, grow your own garlic, or take up affirming activities of your own based on the many examples herein, all part of building your glow with a practice that beautifies your life.

This diverse assortment of categories ensures that through this year's worth of Eat Pretty entries, you'll see your beauty as the sum of its many true parts—your meals, habits, outlook, and intentions—and not the sum of the contents of your bathroom cabinet and your makeup bag. Start making small shifts. Eat new foods and adopt new mindsets. Break the mold that you may have unknowingly fit yourself into. Try some of the ideas in this book on for size, to see how they fit you in turn. When you do, there's no telling how beautiful this year, and you yourself, can become.

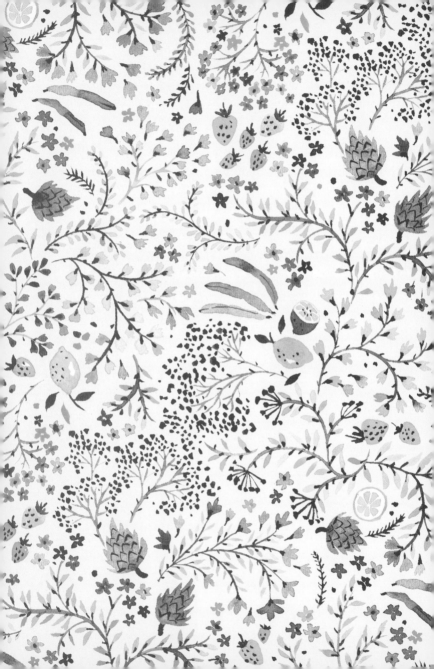

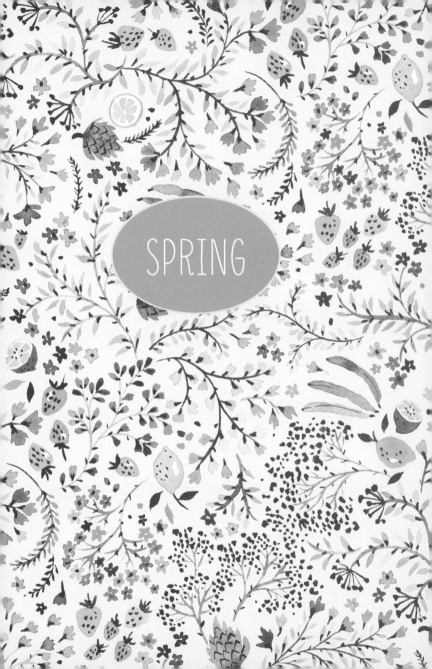

SPRING

Spring is the season of new beginnings. Like the plants coming back to life around you, the renewed energy of your beauty and body burst forth, eager for new challenges and experiences. The chill of winter melts away, leaving you ready for lighter meals that place more emphasis on raw foods, natural detox, shedding winter weight if you've gained it, and a cleansed, pared-down diet and routine that support optimal digestion and elimination.

The more than ninety daily readings in the section ahead will challenge and inspire you to create beautifying moments every day this season. You'll learn to reach for the foods that support your body's inherent detoxification processes, including an abundance of fresh greens like arugula, dandelion, spinach, and watercress, and vegetables like asparagus, artichokes, radishes, and peas. Lemons are an ideal fruit for spring detox and liver support, so you'll be encouraged to start a habit of drinking a glass of warm lemon water each morning. To enhance the detox process, this spring, make a concerted effort to cut back on the Beauty Betrayers you met on page 10. You'll start to see truly radiant skin that appears refreshed, like spring itself.

While you're giving yourself a new start, I'll also encourage you to rethink your routine. Seek out habits that spark your creativity and refresh your mindset, two strategies that will help open you to boundless potential this year. Revive healthy eating and self-care rituals that may have fallen by the wayside over the winter, and reconnect with nature during these lengthening, lightening days. As the spring days pass, embrace the ideas on each new page, even if they feel like things you wouldn't have done in the past.

Your ability to redefine yourself at any moment is one of the most beautiful powers you possess, and this year you're using it to develop a happier, healthier, more energetic, and radiant you. Commit to living like your best self this spring. You can start by turning this page and doing one thing every day that makes you glow.

Living Your Best Life

HOW TO WAKE UP WELL

Some of us dash out of bed and into the day, smartphone in hand, the moment we hear the morning alarm. Others of us press the snooze button three times and drag ourselves into the kitchen, shutting out the world until our first cup of coffee kicks in. Neither of these habits get the day off to an optimal start for our inner and outer beauty and health. Tomorrow, wake up mindfully. After you open your eyes, stay under the covers for a moment. Stretch your limbs, move your toes, and feel your body awaken. Inhale deeply, and think of one joyful, positive thing that could happen in the day ahead. Open the day with possibility and gratitude, and you truly approach the events of the day with different eyes. This slight tweak in your morning routine may sound insignificant, but it creates energy and positivity that will stick with you throughout the day ahead.

Kitchen Inspiration

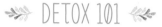 DETOX 101

What's the deal with detox—what is it, exactly? "Detox" is a general name for the processes by which the body removes unwanted and unneeded substances. And here's what we often forget: your body is working hard to detoxify you even as you read this sentence. Detox isn't a food-restricted or liquids-only week you need to schedule on your calendar. But you can help the process by regularly giving your body a break, making simple lifestyle changes that allow your body to detoxify more thoroughly and completely. Here are some simple suggestions. *What to do:* Pack your diet with whole, organic veggies and fruits, healthy fats, and clean proteins and eat only until you're satisfied. Use nontoxic beauty and home cleaning products. Incorporate naturally detoxifying foods like lemons, garlic, turmeric, and asparagus. *What not to do:* Splurge too often on Beauty Betrayers (see page 10), which contain many compounds that your body doesn't need and that won't do any favors for your beauty, either. When you choose to put only the best ingredients in and on your body, detox can be a whole lot simpler— and more delicious—than a restriction-filled cleanse.

Beauty Science

DIET AND ACNE

Think your diet has no effect on the clarity of your skin? Think again. One foundational study on the diet-acne link pointed out that diet *directly influences* several of the primary factors in acne formation, including inflammation, sebum production, and cell turnover. This study also named several populations—including Eskimo and Okinawa islander—with unique diets that show no incidence of acne whatsoever, demonstrating that diet and lifestyle, in addition to genetic factors, are keys to understanding the true cause of our breakouts. Recent studies continue to support the strong diet-acne link, so it's essential to consider your diet if you struggle with blemishes. Sustain your skin and support a clear complexion by eating fresh, whole foods, including healthy fats, clean proteins, and an abundance of colorful veggies this spring and beyond.

Intention of the Week

EAT AT LEAST ONE SERVING OF GREENS EACH DAY

Ready for a visible skin upgrade? Challenge yourself to eat at least one serving (equal to about a medium-sized handful) of greens every day. Take your pick from the many easy and delicious ways to meet this challenge. You can sauté beet greens, crisp up kale chips, blend yourself a dandelion green smoothie, or toss fresh chard into a homemade soup. Hungry for another serving? Go ahead—and give yourself bonus beauty points every time you opt for greens. Since it's spring, the season of greens, explore varieties that might be unfamiliar to you, such as antioxidant-packed bok choy and tatsoi, detoxifying broccoli leaves, or anti-inflammatory mâche, and you'll score big as well. The multitude of skin benefits in even one serving of fresh greens includes a megadose of vitamin A (a powerful skin healer and smoother that prevents blemishes and UV damage), vitamin C, essential beauty minerals like iron, and dark circle–busting vitamin K. Complete this greens-a-day challenge, and you'll most assuredly notice more energy and a more radiant-looking complexion in the mirror. Oh, and you'll start a key beautifying habit that may stick long after the week is over!

Time for Self-Love

STAY FLEXIBLE

Resilience defines our ability to age well, both inside and out. We can maximize the physical resilience of our skin day to day by choosing nourishing foods and lifestyle habits, and we can maximize the resilience of our spirits by learning to manage our emotional ups and downs. In doing so, we become better able to handle the inevitable stresses, changes, and unexpected twists of life. Today, build your resilience by gracefully receiving whatever comes your way; this conscious act supports lifelong beauty, inside and out.

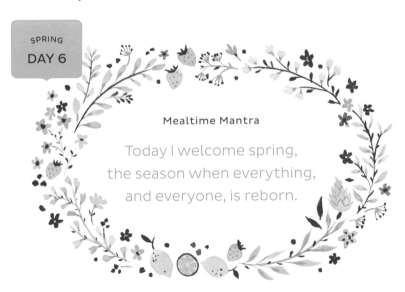

Mealtime Mantra

Today I welcome spring,
the season when everything,
and everyone, is reborn.

Eat Pretty Recipe

WEEKDAY BREAKFAST DONE RIGHT

SHIITAKE-HERB SCRAMBLE

Even just ten minutes in the kitchen can produce a breakfast that keeps you energized throughout the morning—if it's made with the right ingredients. The complex flavor of shiitake mushrooms, one of my favorite energy foods, along with an abundance of antioxidant-rich herbs make this simple breakfast truly satisfying. Substitute any fresh, savory herbs you have on hand (try chives, thyme, dill, or basil), and multiply the ingredients to serve a family.

SERVES 1

1 tsp coconut oil or grass-fed organic butter

2 oz (55 g) shiitake mushroom caps (about 2 handfuls), brushed clean and roughly chopped

2 pastured eggs (see page 248), beaten

1 Tbsp chopped fresh parsley

1 tsp minced fresh sage

1 or 2 pinches ground turmeric

Unrefined salt and freshly ground black pepper

Melt the coconut oil or butter in a skillet over medium heat. Add the mushrooms and sauté until tender and reduced, about 5 minutes. Pour the eggs over the mushrooms and sprinkle with the herbs and turmeric. Cook, stirring gently once or twice to distribute the herbs and move the uncooked portion of egg underneath, until set, about 2 minutes longer. Season with salt and pepper. Serve immediately.

Beauty Food Profile

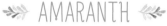

AMARANTH

Ounce for ounce, this tiny grain, which gets quite sticky when cooked, packs more calcium than milk. This calcium comes packaged for optimal absorption with a powerful lineup of amino acids that also strengthen bones and collagen. In addition to calcium, amaranth grains (which are technically seeds) offer a range of powerful beauty minerals that support bones, hair, and skin, including manganese for healthy hair and hair color and iron for energy. And as a foundation to it all, amaranth contains about 8 g of beautifying protein, essential for building and maintaining your beauty, in just ¼ cup [50 g]. Cook it into a creamy breakfast cereal, toss cooked amaranth with greens and veggies to supercharge a salad, or heat the seeds in a skillet until they pop into an addictive snack.

EAT PRETTY FOOD	BEAUTIFYING COMPOUND	BEAUTY BENEFIT
Amaranth	Calcium	Strengthens teeth, bones, and nails

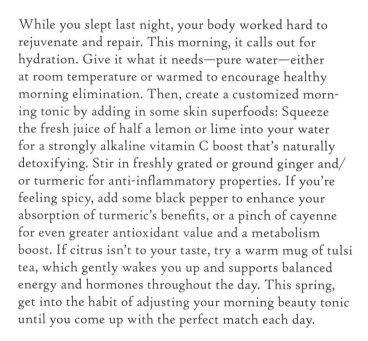

Kitchen Inspiration

MAKE A MORNING BEAUTY TONIC

While you slept last night, your body worked hard to rejuvenate and repair. This morning, it calls out for hydration. Give it what it needs—pure water—either at room temperature or warmed to encourage healthy morning elimination. Then, create a customized morning tonic by adding in some skin superfoods: Squeeze the fresh juice of half a lemon or lime into your water for a strongly alkaline vitamin C boost that's naturally detoxifying. Stir in freshly grated or ground ginger and/or turmeric for anti-inflammatory properties. If you're feeling spicy, add some black pepper to enhance your absorption of turmeric's benefits, or a pinch of cayenne for even greater antioxidant value and a metabolism boost. If citrus isn't to your taste, try a warm mug of tulsi tea, which gently wakes you up and supports balanced energy and hormones throughout the day. This spring, get into the habit of adjusting your morning beauty tonic until you come up with the perfect match each day.

Time for Self-Love

SEE SELF-LOVE AS ESSENTIAL

In our busy lives, it's easy to put off self-care activities. But taking time to love yourself is essential, like sleeping and eating well. Self-care allows you to look, feel, and perform at your best each and every day, and you'll be noticeably more radiant when you apply it regularly. If you get stuck coming up with healthy and beautifying ways to love and care for yourself, simply give yourself the gift of time to think, daydream, and plan a life that feels true to you. Ask yourself what you need on this day, or at this moment in your life, and find healthy, beautifying ways to meet those changing needs. Think of your time for self-love as a vital piece of your daily nourishment and you'll increase both your beauty and your happiness.

Pretty Pairing
PISTACHIOS + FIGS

Why they're more beautiful together: This decadent pairing works together in taste and function. Vitamin B_6 in pistachios helps the body to better absorb calming magnesium found in figs. Together B_6 and magnesium support rejuvenating sleep, stress reduction, and healthy nervous function.

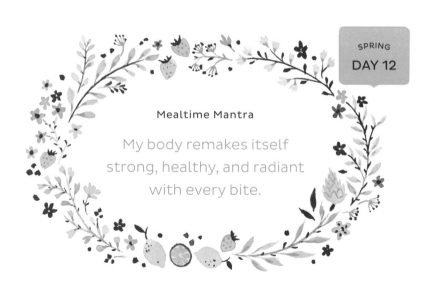

Mealtime Mantra

My body remakes itself
strong, healthy, and radiant
with every bite.

Intention of the Week

SWAP IN GREEN BEAUTY PRODUCTS

Safe personal care products are an incredibly important aspect of your lifelong beauty and health, as they have major influence on your chemical exposures and hormonal balance. If you haven't yet turned over the label to get a closer look at what's in the products you use every day, start now. To make the biggest impact on your health with the least amount of effort, pick one of the products you use most regularly, like a deodorant you wear daily or a lipstick you apply and reapply each day, or something you apply over a large surface area of your body, like a body lotion that you slather on head to toe. Make sure your formula is free of some of the most consistent offenders: hormone-disrupting parabens and phthalates; antibacterial compounds like triclosan; synthetic colors, fragrances and dyes; and chemical sunscreens, like oxybenzone. If you spot some of these ingredients, replace the product with one displaying a certified organic seal on the packaging, or made with ingredients you recognize—like shea butter, coconut oil, or green tea. You'll be detoxing your body simply by reducing the amount of chemicals you take in each day. How quickly can detox take place inside your body? One recent study showed that women who switched their conventional personal care products to natural versions experienced a 27 to 45 percent reduction in levels of potentially harmful ingredients like parabens, phthalates, triclosan, and oxybenzone in their urine after just three days.

Living Your Best Life

HOW TO INSTANTLY IMPROVE THE AIR QUALITY IN YOUR HOME

Breathe in deeply, hold the breath for a moment, then let it out. Clean air is an overlooked beauty must-have; it's the body's most basic nutrient-delivery system and a powerful waste eliminator. So what kind of air are you breathing? Indoor air quality in our homes is often poor due to fragrances from things like candles and cleaning supplies; off-gases from paint and varnishes, furniture, and carpets; and fireplace smoke—especially after a long winter, when little outside air enters. Today, open windows that have been shuttered for months and allow fresh air to cycle in. And, while the hot-weather months are still only looming, opt for fresh-air breezes through your home rather than switching directly from heat to air conditioning. Do the same with your lungs by exercising outdoors, where nature now blooms with air-purifying green plants. You'll support beautifying detox by delivering fresh air into your system, whether you're inside or out.

Beauty Food Profile

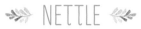 NETTLE

Nettle, a leafy green that looks similar to mint, is an alkaline herbal powerhouse for beauty and detox. Nettles contain high concentrations of key minerals—including calcium, iron, silicon, and magnesium—that support healthy hair, nails, bones, and skin. In the spring, you may find young nettle leaves at farmers' markets, ready for steaming and eating, and in-the-know foragers will find them in the wild (they bring along gloves to avoid touching stinging nettle leaves), where they're often collected for exclusive restaurants. By far the easiest way for most of us to get our nettle is to sip organic nettle tea, which offers some of the same mineral-rich, anti-histamine, water retention–reducing, and blood sugar-lowering beauty benefits as the fresh leaf.

EAT PRETTY FOOD	BEAUTIFYING COMPOUND	BEAUTY BENEFIT
Nettle	Silicon	Strengthens skin and hair

Time for Self-Love

DIGEST WITH YOGA

We know that yoga can improve our flexibility and focus—but did you know it can also aid in digestion? Practicing yoga after a meal—even just a few poses—can bring circulation to your core, where digestion takes place. It can also relieve gas and bloating, and give an internal massage to your organs that support elimination. Give the following short sequence a try after an upcoming meal. Do it slowly, and take five deep, long breaths every time you change position. Start by lying back on the floor with your knees bent and your arms at your sides. Let your knees fall to the left while your head and arms stretch toward the right. Return to center and switch sides, lowering your knees to the right and turning your head and arms to the left. Return to center and hug your knees to your chest, rocking side to side gently. Sit up and cross your left leg over your right, bending your knee to keep your left foot on the floor. Twist your body to the left, hold, and breathe. Repeat on the opposite side.

Kitchen Inspiration
❧ SPRING SMOOTHIE ADD-INS ❧

Want to target the needs of your beauty and body with a smoothie that's tailored to spring beauty? To maximize detox, support natural cleansing, and supercharge your beauty after a long winter, try these superfood smoothie add-ins: flaxseed, for fiber and detox (try 2 Tbsp in a smoothie); spirulina, for energy and beauty minerals (start with 1 tsp for a nutrient boost); and matcha tea powder, for concentrated antioxidants and energy (matcha also contains caffeine, so use only ¼ to 1 tsp, depending on your caffeine tolerance).

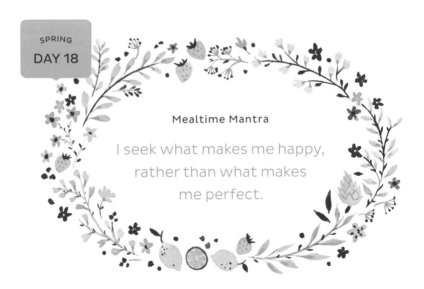

Mealtime Mantra

I seek what makes me happy, rather than what makes me perfect.

Time for Self-Love
REFRESH YOUR SCALP

We spend an overwhelming amount of time caring for the skin on our face, feet, legs, hands, and arms, but we often ignore the skin on our scalp. A healthy scalp supports your strongest, most beautiful hair, so a little extra attention to the skin up there gives an easy beauty and self-care boost. Cleansing and massaging your scalp helps remove dead skin cells and increase scalp circulation to deliver nourishment, stimulate hair follicles, and distribute natural oils that keep your hair shiny and healthy. It also lights up the sensitive nerves on your scalp and reduces tension (head massage, anyone?). As an occasional scalp treatment, generously apply a natural hair and scalp oil to your fingers and gently massage into your scalp. Or make your own blend using scalp-friendly oils like neem and coconut. Leave the oils on for half an hour or more, then shampoo thoroughly.

Intention of the Week

LISTEN TO YOUR SKIN

While it may be frustrating to wake up to a huge pimple, to battle dry patches and flare-ups of eczema or rashes, and to feel like your skin is just plain lackluster at times, remember that these unwanted skin states aren't simply cropping up because you lost the flawless-skin lottery. They are signs. Your skin is a direct reflection of the inner health of your body—hence your efforts to Eat Pretty Every Day. But there will be times when your inner health gets off balance, whether from stress, illness, dietary choices that don't agree with you, or other life-style factors. At those times, expect that your skin will be one of the first pointers to tell you when you've gone too far off track. This week, practice using your skin as a window to your inner health. If you see signs of redness and inflammation or a random breakout, ask yourself if a recent food or habit could be the catalyst. If your skin looks brighter and more glowing than usual, think for a moment if you can attribute it to a healthy new practice. Looking to your skin as a barometer of your inner health helps you stay closely connected with your body and take ownership of your beauty, head to toe.

Eat Pretty Recipe

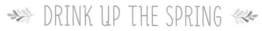

DRINK UP THE SPRING

LATE SPRING STRAWBERRY BASIL LEMONADE

In spring, it's best to eat sweet fruits in moderation, since it's the time of year when we're detoxing and lightening with lots of green veggies and very little sugar. But how can we resist juicy fruits like newly ripened strawberries? The collagen-building vitamin C in these bright berries makes it more than okay to indulge. The tart, alkaline lemon and anti-inflammatory basil in this beautifying sip combine to make it a savory-sweet alternative to lemon water.

SERVES 4 OR 5

4 cups [960 ml] purified water
2 cups [240 g] organic
  strawberries, hulled
1 organic lemon, peeled, halved,
  and seeded

½ cup [15 g] loosely packed fresh
  basil leaves
4 drops liquid stevia

In a high-powered blender, combine all of the ingredients and process until smooth, about 60 seconds. If desired, strain the lemonade through a fine-mesh sieve before serving at room temperature or over ice.

Kitchen Inspiration

✤ DRESS UP SALAD ✤

Although they're convenient, store-bought salad dressings are a sneaky source of beauty-betraying ingredients like processed oils, added sugars, synthetic colors, and undesirable preservatives. It only takes a tiny amount of effort to perfect your own repertoire of quick homemade dressings—and it's fun to get creative with flavors and beautifying add-ins once you've developed this skill. The next time you sit down to a salad, dress it up with a skin-friendly vinaigrette: Start with a mix of acid (lemon juice, lime juice, apple cider vinegar, and balsamic vinegar are favorites) and oil (extra-virgin olive oil is the perennial favorite, but try sesame, flax, or hemp as well). You can go 50/50 with your acid/oil mix, or use the time-tested 1:3 acid-to-oil ratio. Season with unrefined salt and freshly ground pepper, and then add flavor with herbs, spices, and other aromatics—minced fresh garlic; fresh or dried herbs like oregano and dill; hot, sweet, or dry mustard; grated fresh ginger; and chopped shallot or scallion are delicious in varying combos. Whisk the ingredients together in a bowl or shake them up in a jar, and you have an instant classic. Remember: oils like olive oil solidify in the fridge, so if you store leftover dressing, take it out of the refrigerator at least ten minutes before you want to use it.

Beauty Science

HAPPY, AND HEALTHY, MEALS AT HOME

Want to eat healthier at home? Then make your house or apartment a sacred, aesthetically pleasing space. One study found that feeling positive emotions at home triggered healthier food choices—which in turn triggered even more positive emotions (no surprise there; we already know that beauty food leaves us feeling uplifted!). To initiate this beautifying cycle in your own life, try sprucing up your kitchen space, paring down mess and clutter, or—in celebration of springtime— bringing inside blossoming flowers.

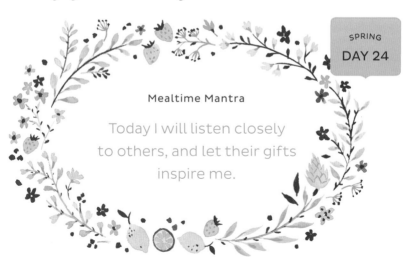

Mealtime Mantra

Today I will listen closely to others, and let their gifts inspire me.

Living Your Best Life

HOW TO CREATE SPACE FOR YOUR BEST SELF

In the spirit of renewal that comes with spring, use this season to pare down in your home and your daily routine. Excess—whether in eating, demands on your time, or possessions—weighs down your body, mind, and spirit. Pick one area of your life that feels overwhelming or disorganized, like your spice cabinet, your work or social calendar, or your makeup bag, and weed through it. Get rid of anything that's extraneous, outdated, expired, or went unused in the last year. And if you come across something that just doesn't align with your current health and beauty goals, toss that too. You'll free up valuable energy and space that can be put toward the thoughtful curation of belongings—including healthier foods—that reflect your best self in mind, body, and spirit.

Beauty Food Profile

❧ RAW HONEY ❧

Honey is a unique natural sweetener with benefits well beyond its concentrated sweetness. Raw honey contains beneficial enzymes and nutrients as well as bee pollen, a complete protein, and bee propolis, a substance with anti-viral and antibiotic properties. Raw honey is an alkaline food that has antibacterial qualities, attributed in scientific study to its natural content of hydrogen peroxide, its low pH, and a unique protein made by bees called defensin-1. Raw honey's antibacterial benefits support inner health, as well as outer healing of the skin, including cuts and blemishes. Its demulcent properties make it a soother of coughs and sore throats. Be sure to purchase honey that's labeled "raw," or labeled as unheated and unpasteurized, as much of the conventional honey stocked in stores is highly processed and devoid of the enzymes, pollen, and nutrients that make raw honey so exceptional. If you're lucky enough to get your hands on raw Manuka honey, which is made with pollen from the medicinal Manuka plant, you'll have an even more powerful healer with mighty antibacterial properties. Raw honey keeps indefinitely, so it's an ideal pantry item.

EAT PRETTY FOOD	BEAUTIFYING COMPOUND	BEAUTY BENEFIT
Raw honey	Defensin-1 protein	Antibacterial

Kitchen Inspiration

EAT FOR A GLUTATHIONE BOOST

Glutathione is the body's master antioxidant, one that has the power to slow aging by regenerating the anti-oxidant vitamins C and E in the body, detoxifying, and supporting immunity and the health and function of your mitochondria. Maintaining high levels of glutathione is one of the most important things we can do to promote beautiful aging. But all kinds of everyday stressors, from injuries and infections to the negative effects of prescription drugs and processed foods, deplete it. So you'll be happy to know that you can support glutathione production in your body with beauty food! Foods that stimulate glutathione production include the entire category of sulfur-rich brassica vegetables, especially broccoli sprouts, as well as onions, spinach, asparagus, avocados, turmeric, garlic, beets, Brazil nuts, and even watermelon rind. Foods rich in vitamin C, selenium, and alpha-lipoic acid, like spinach, beets, and sunflower seeds, help this process as well. Fill your kitchen with these foods and feast on them regularly for natural detox and powerful beauty support.

Time for Self-Love
⤜ SET YOUR MIND ON BEAUTY ⤛

Your mind is a powerful thing. It influences digestion, healing, and even your outward appearance. Don't take it from me; look to the budding field of psychodermatology for proof! The close connectedness of the skin and the brain means that we can observe physical reactions (like flushing, itching, blemishes, and rashes) that are directly influenced by emotional states. I strongly believe that our emotions can be harnessed for positive beauty benefits through that very same connection. Liken it to the placebo effect: when you believe that you are getting better, you often do. Believe that you are beautiful, that your skin is radiant, and that you are your best version of yourself today, and you *are*. This spring, adjust your mindset, or simply find more things you love about yourself, for an untapped beauty boost.

Intention of the Week
DRINK WARM LEMON WATER EVERY MORNING

For a simple practice that will start your day off beautifully seven days a week, squeeze the juice of half a lemon into a mug of warm (not boiling) water and sip first thing in the morning. Lemon juice is a beauty powerhouse that delivers a collagen-building, antioxidant-packed vitamin C boost while supporting the liver cleansing, detox, and elimination essential to glowing skin. It also has a highly alkaline effect inside the body, which balances excess acidity from foods like dairy, sugar, and meat. Keep the a.m. habit going to see brighter, more radiant, better-hydrated skin over time.

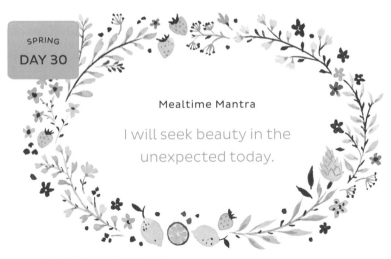

Mealtime Mantra

I will seek beauty in the unexpected today.

Beauty Science

THE ROOT OF ALL HAPPINESS

On the surface, happiness is pretty simple: a feeling of well-being, pleasure, and contentment, and a sense that all is right with the world. But one recent study found that the *source* of your happiness can influence your overall health—in a way that also impacts your beauty and aging. Two types of happiness were studied: hedonic well-being, or the happiness that comes from self-gratification (think, having cool stuff or experiences), and eudaimonic well-being, or the happiness that comes from having a greater sense of purpose in life (think, a career or volunteering work that leaves you feeling fulfilled). As you might guess, those who felt high levels of eudaimonic well-being benefited more, displaying low levels of inflammatory gene expression and strong expression of antiviral and antibody genes. Those who showed high levels of hedonic well-being actually had high inflammatory gene expression, as well as low antiviral and antibody gene expression. With inflammation so closely tied to health, beauty, and longevity, the takeaway is profound: finding happiness in a meaningful life is measurably better for your health and beauty than finding happiness in material pleasures.

Eat Pretty Recipe

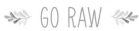 GO RAW

SPRINGTIME SUMMER ROLLS
WITH SWEET RED CURRY DIPPING SAUCE

This light meal, packed with healthy fats and detoxifying vege-
tables, is an easy way to enjoy the beauty benefits of raw foods.
Let the antioxidant-packed dipping sauce make each bite satis-
fying and special.

MAKES 8 ROLLS

¼ cup [55 g] tahini
2 Tbsp unsweetened non-dairy
  milk
1 Tbsp maple syrup
4 tsp red curry paste
2 tsp low-sodium, wheat-free
  tamari
Eight 6-in [15-cm] rice paper
  wrappers

1 ripe avocado, pitted, peeled,
  and cut into 16 wedges
8 large fresh basil leaves
8 raw slender asparagus spears,
  tough ends removed
4 cups [120 g] packed arugula or
  watercress

To make the dipping sauce, in a small serving bowl,
whisk together the tahini, milk, maple syrup, curry paste,
and tamari. Set aside.

Working with one rice paper at a time, assemble the
rolls: Dip a wrapper briefly in a shallow bowl of warm
water, dab off the excess moisture on a clean kitchen towel,
and lay it flat on a work surface. Fill with 2 wedges of
avocado, a basil leaf torn into pieces, a stalk of asparagus
broken into thirds, and ½ cup greens. Fold in the sides of
wrapper, then fold up the bottom and roll into a tight cyl-
inder. Repeat to make the remaining rolls. Serve with the
dipping sauce.

Time for Self-Love

BRUSH YOUR WAY TO BETTER SKIN

Lymph, a detoxifying, nutrient-delivering fluid that flows just beneath your skin, is an underappreciated beauty booster and support system for your beautifying diet, since it delivers nutrition to your cells and shuttles away waste. A wonderful self-care technique called "dry brushing" encourages the circulation of lymph, which slows due to lack of exercise (including too much time spent sitting, which many of us are prone to in winter), inflammation, stress, poor diet, and even surgery, resulting in visible puffiness, dull skin, dark circles, and water retention. To get your lymph moving and improve the tone, texture, and health of your skin this spring, set aside time for a regular dry-brushing session.

To dry brush, all you need is a stiff-bristled body brush, which you can find in a well-stocked pharmacy, beauty supply store, or online. I recommend brushing after bathing, when your skin is clean and dry. Brush your naked body with gentle yet stimulating strokes, working from your feet up your calves and thighs, and toward your heart. You'll feel your skin tingle immediately, signaling a circulation boost. Follow this calming ritual with your favorite natural body oil or lotion, massaging it into the skin in the same direction—upward, working in toward your heart. Dry brush at least once a week for softer, healthier skin that you'll be proud to bare.

Kitchen Inspiration

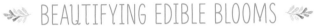 BEAUTIFYING EDIBLE BLOOMS

When you plant your garden this season, expand your crop of edible beauty foods into the floral realm. Several easily grown varieties of flowering plants are not only edible but also brimming with antioxidant phytochemicals that support gorgeous skin. A recent study found that extracts of ten common edible flowers, from Chinese roses to chrysanthemums, are full of anti-inflammatory antioxidants. The most antioxidant-rich edible flower in the study came from the tree peony, but the common honeysuckle flower also rated highly. Other edible flowering plants you might want to include in your garden are nasturtium and French lavender. Be careful to choose the correct edible varieties and be sure they are pesticide-free, then sprinkle their blooms liberally on your salads and desserts this spring for visually stunning beauty benefits.

Pretty Pairing

✻ MATCHA TEA + GRAPEFRUIT ✻

Why they're more beautiful together: Matcha green tea
alone is a fabulous sip for beauty thanks to its incredibly
high antioxidant content, which includes the phytochemical EGCG that interrupts part of the skin-wrinkling
process. Enjoy matcha tea with a squeeze of grapefruit
juice or a wedge of grapefruit, however, and your body
will reap far more antioxidant benefits, since citrus
juice allows the body to absorb even more of green tea's
powerful anti-aging compounds.

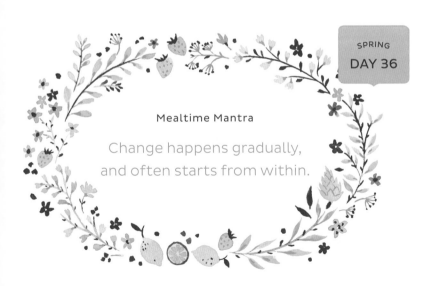

Mealtime Mantra

Change happens gradually,
and often starts from within.

Beauty Food Profile

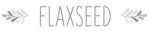 FLAXSEED

Flaxseed is a top-notch beauty booster to add to your morning smoothie or cereal—just make sure you grind the seeds to allow their nutrients to be better absorbed. Flaxseed contains alpha-linolenic acid, which the body converts to skin-friendly, anti-inflammatory omega-3s that are essential for gorgeous, youthful skin. Flaxseed may also protect against oxidative damage by strengthening cells' natural defenses. Its mucilaginous properties (it forms a sticky gel when soaked in water, which is why flax is a frequently used binding substitute in egg-free baked goods) can soothe intestinal issues and detoxify, and its fiber encourages healthy elimination. Flaxseed is also a source of lignans, phytoestrogens that help to regulate estrogen levels in the body. Store your seeds in an airtight container in the refrigerator to preserve their delicate oils.

EAT PRETTY FOOD	BEAUTIFYING COMPOUND	BEAUTY BENEFIT
Flaxseed	Alpha-linolenic acid	Reduces inflammation

Intention of the Week

EAT A BEAUTIFYING BREAKFAST EVERY DAY

Breakfast: It truly is the most important meal of the day. It sets the tone for the way you'll eat and feel all day, even as it keeps your blood sugar stable and your energy up— that is, if you choose well. What makes for a great beauty breakfast? A dose of clean protein, healthy fats, and anti-oxidant-rich veggies and fruits. Today, try a pastured egg scramble with vegetables and herbs (see page 29); a smoothie packed with greens, avocado, and protein-rich hemp seeds; or cinnamon-spiced oatmeal with colorful berries and a spoonful of almond butter stirred in. What happens if you skip breakfast, or grab something less beautifying? Don't feel as if you've failed for the entire day. But tomorrow and going forward, see your a.m. meal for its beauty potential, and continue striving to set the tone for looking and feeling your best first thing in the morning.

Living Your Best Life
REAP THE BEAUTY BENEFITS OF A GARDEN

If you haven't yet had the time or circumstances to grow your own food, from seed to sprout to flourishing plant, take this day, this season, to get a project underway. The beauty benefits of homegrown are threefold: Getting your hands in the dirt and connecting with the earth dramatically lowers stress. Planting something edible—say, cucumbers or parsley—means you'll be able to reap the nutritional beauty benefits, which are potent in freshly picked food, by simply eating your creations. Last but not least, your exposure to tiny soil-based organisms, both on the food you grow and in the soil you come into contact with, helps to defend against bad bacteria and round out a thriving microbiome, the population of bacteria that live in and on your body. If you find yourself limited by time or space constraints, even a windowsill garden in your kitchen does the trick. For your beauty, any one of these benefits is reason enough to get growing today.

Kitchen Inspiration

LET GARLIC REST

You'll get more beauty benefits from your fresh garlic if you chop, mince, or otherwise crush it, then let it hang out for ten or fifteen minutes before using it in your cooking. Here's the science behind this tip, as reported in one fascinating study: crushing garlic sets in motion a process that forms allicin, a phytochemical that helps reduce inflammation and slow the breakdown of collagen. The study found that letting crushed garlic rest for ten minutes before cooking with it enhanced the formation of allicin even further. So chop your garlic first, and then let it charge up its content of beauty-boosting phytochemicals without any extra work on your part! Since heat degrades many of the protective benefits of garlic, letting crushed cloves stand and then cooking them lightly helps retain as many anti-aging compounds as possible.

Beauty Science

BUILD BEAUTIFUL BONES

Recent research shows that vitamin K_2—which is often lacking in our diets, and which is found in some fermented foods, egg yolks, and grass-fed butter—has major bone-building benefits. Vitamin K_2 works with vitamin D to help deposit calcium in our bones and teeth, and has even been found to strengthen bone density in women who have osteoporosis. Just one key reason to get K_2-rich foods in your beautifying diet regularly.

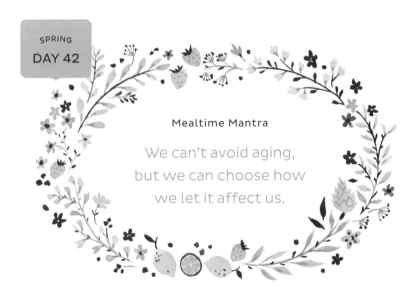

Mealtime Mantra

We can't avoid aging, but we can choose how we let it affect us.

Time for Self-Love

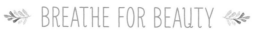 BREATHE FOR BEAUTY

Open your mind to pranayama, a breathing practice that helps deepen your beauty and balance your hormones. The name unites the Sanskrit words *prana*, for "vital energy" or "life force," and *yama*, meaning to "extend" or "draw out." And just think: "extending life force" is another way of saying "aging beautifully"!

One of my favorite pranayama exercises is Alternate Nostril Breathing, a well-known breath exercise with instant stress-lowering benefits. To practice, breathe in through one nostril and out through the other—always closing off the opposite nostril with a finger. Then repeat, switching to inhale through the other nostril. Start with five minutes and work your way up to fifteen. This practice not only allows me to get a handle on rising stress, it gives me a fallback relaxation technique for moments of anxiety that might otherwise push me to panic. Try this technique to see if it becomes one your own tools for relaxation, or explore other pranayama breaths to find your favorite.

Intention of the Week

MAKE TIME TO JOURNAL EVERY DAY

The practice of journaling has been shown to reduce stress, help you get better beauty sleep, and improve your mood and mental clarity—all important aspects of looking and feeling your best. If you aren't a regular journal writer, try the practice this week to see if you appreciate the benefits in your life. If journaling in the morning, your daily journal entry might be a one-line intention for the day ahead, or if journaling at night, you might create a list of bullet points that help you organize random thoughts before bed. If you want to write more than a simple line or list, go for it. You may find that your best ideas—and most peaceful nights of sleep—emerge from a journaling session.

Eat Pretty Recipe

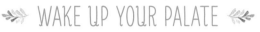

WAKE UP YOUR PALATE

DETOXIFYING ASPARAGUS SPEARS
WITH CREAMY SCALLION DIP

Asparagus boosts the anti-aging, detoxifying antioxidant glutathione in your body, but when we cook it (and, too often, overcook it), it loses some of its most beautifying nutrition. Raw asparagus has a satisfying snap and a savory depth that pairs well with this creamy dip, packed with its own dose of detoxifying, collagen-protecting phytochemicals and skin-clearing zinc.

SERVES 4 TO 6

1 tsp plus 1 Tbsp coconut oil
3 scallions, white and crisp green parts only, chopped
1 shallot, finely chopped
½ cup [60 g] raw cashews, soaked in water for at least 4 hours or overnight, drained and rinsed

1 cup [100 g] cooked white beans
⅛ tsp unrefined salt
¼ cup [60 ml] fresh lemon juice
1 bunch organic asparagus, tough ends removed

In a small sauté pan or skillet, melt the 1 tsp coconut oil over medium heat. Add the scallions and shallot, reserving 2 tsp of the chopped scallion greens, and sauté until soft and golden, about 5 minutes. Remove from the heat. In a high-powered blender or food processor, combine the cashews, the 1 Tbsp coconut oil, the cooked scallions and shallot, the beans, the reserved raw scallion greens, the salt, and the lemon juice. Process until the dip is creamy and free of any lumps, about 5 minutes, pausing frequently to scrape down the sides of the blender or food processor. Serve at room temperature with the raw asparagus spears for dipping.

Beauty Food Profile

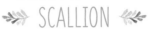 SCALLION

The scallion is one of the alliums, a family of anti-inflammatory foods (including leeks, garlic, onions, and ramps) that are staples for gorgeous skin and a healthy immune system. Allicin, a phytochemical found in scallions, helps preserve youthful collagen and prevent signs of aging by protecting a powerful enzyme in the body that stops the action of other collagen-digesting, wrinkle-forming enzymes. Just a few tablespoons of chopped scallions contains over 70 percent of your RDA of vitamin K_1, a blood vessel strengthener, so eat up to keep capillaries strong and prevent dark circles and bruising. The supercharged combo of beta-carotene, lutein, and zeaxanthin in scallions also maintains youthful eyesight.

EAT PRETTY FOOD	BEAUTIFYING COMPOUND	BEAUTY BENEFIT
Scallion	Allicin	Protects collagen

Kitchen Inspiration

THE SURPRISING BEAUTY BENEFITS OF BITTERS

Hiding among the liquor bottles in your cocktail bar is a surprisingly beauty-friendly liquid: bitters. Sipped on its own, this herbal brew (made from various combinations of bitter herbs) can jumpstart your digestion. Bitters signal your body to secrete digestive enzymes that support more effective breakdown of food, and strengthen your digestive organs over time. Just a few drops of bitters on your tongue or added to a small amount of water, taken fifteen minutes before a meal, start that healthy process. For best-quality bitters, look for certified organic brews.

Time for Self-Love

✵ BUILD UP YOUR OJAS ✵

In Ayurvedic teachings, one by-product of healthy digestion is a powerfully beautifying essence called *ojas* (pronounced "oh-jus"). You might not have heard the term, but you are definitely familiar with its effects. Ojas produces a state of optimal physical health that we see on the outside as glow, vibrancy, and radiant beauty. I love this concept because it puts into words the beauty that we all seek, inside and out. If you're still struggling to see or feed your own radiance, then ojas, with its connotations of perfection, may seem unattainable. But just think: the fact that it is connected to digestion means that every one of us can strive for it by nourishing a healthy digestive system. To do that, we eat healthy, whole foods, including those rich in probiotics, and prioritize self-care, from exercise to healthy beauty rituals and sleep. In doing so, we can build up our ojas and uncover that vibrant, sought-after state of beauty in the process.

Living Your Best Life

HOW TO DRAW A SPA-WORTHY BATH

A bath can be far more than a simple soak in water. Add any number of beautifying enhancers and you'll easily benefit from a spa-worthy bath in your own home. Epsom salts soothe sore, tired muscles and increase your levels of magnesium, the beauty mineral that relaxes the body and prepares you for restful sleep. Dead Sea salts also boost magnesium while lowering inflammation and improving the hydration and softness of your skin. Don't have any bath salts? Add a sprinkle of baking soda to your bath for an all-natural skin softener. Skip bubble baths with synthetic fragrances or skin-drying chemicals and opt for essential oils instead, which are far more therapeutic for your body and senses. A few favorite essential oils for soaking are lavender for relaxation and calm, rose for stress relief, ylang-ylang for restful sleep and well-being, and juniper for detox and energy. Let the scent of the oil fill the warm air around you; breathing in the fragrant oils is part of this all-senses experience.

Kitchen Inspiration

TRY NEW PRODUCE

That vegetables are having a renaissance in homes and restaurants around the world means new varieties are being cultivated—sometimes from heirloom seeds that have been saved for decades—and popping up at markets all the time. Keep your eyes open and you'll frequently find new produce that you've *never seen or tasted before.* Look out for fiddleheads in the spring, Romanesco broccoli in the summer, and honeynut squash in the fall. When you see a new type of vegetable or fruit, by all means—try it! Don't wait until you have a recipe or read that it's trendy. If it's fresh and organic, you can be absolutely certain that it has unique beauty benefits. Getting passionate about new varieties of vegetables may even keep your eyes from wandering toward the splashy packages of cookies and processed snacks at the grocery store. Often there are far more interesting things to see in the produce aisle. Bottom line: you can expand your palate with new flavors and taste combinations without having to reach for a taste that's artificial.

Intention of the Week

DITCH PROCESSED FOODS FOR WHOLE FOODS

Sure, going all whole food, all the time, is next to impossible in our convenience-filled lives. But try it for one week, and you might find that it's easier than you think—and that your efforts will be noticeable in the mirror. Unlike processed foods, whole foods are exactly like (or very near to) their natural state, like a potato (not a chip) or a handful of raspberries (not raspberry fruit snacks). The beauty benefits of bringing more whole foods into your diet cannot be overstated. When you eat whole foods, you receive complementary nutrients that work together to support optimal health and beauty. When you eat whole foods, you avoid added colors, flavors, and preservatives. And when you eat whole foods, you give your body tools it knows how to use to defend, repair, and detox your beauty from the inside out. Skip the processed foods this week (get your groceries from a farmers' market to make this intention easier to commit to) and see how much more you glow.

Pretty Pairing

BROWN RICE +
APPLE CIDER VINEGAR

Why they're more beautiful together: Having rice? Whip up a quick dressing of apple cider vinegar (ACV) and olive oil, and drizzle it on top before serving. Probiotic-rich ACV livens up the earthy flavor of brown rice, plus the pairing has been shown to make you feel more satisfied after eating and reduce the spike in blood sugar from eating carbohydrate-heavy rice—by an impressive 25 percent.

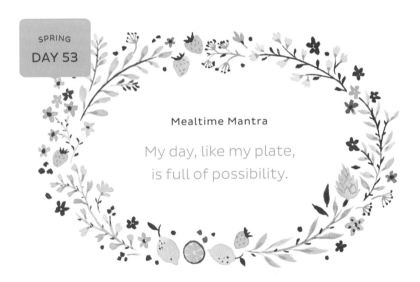

Mealtime Mantra

My day, like my plate,
is full of possibility.

Beauty Food Profile

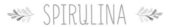 SPIRULINA

For a super-potent, super-green smoothie booster, check out spirulina, a powdered form of blue-green algae. Spirulina is a popular energizer due to its high content of amino acids, making it a complete protein source. Spirulina contains eighteen amino acids, including tryptophan, which our bodies use to make the feel-good neurotransmitter serotonin. One tablespoon (7 g) of nutrient-dense spirulina contains about 4 g of protein and 11 percent of your daily iron intake. Spirulina is alkalizing, contains detoxifying chlorophyll, and is also a good source of sulfur, an important healthy hair nutrient. Always look for high-quality spirulina that's been tested to be sure that it's free of heavy metals and contamination.

EAT PRETTY FOOD	BEAUTIFYING COMPOUND	BEAUTY BENEFIT
Spirulina	Protein	Aids in cell growth and repair

Eat Pretty Recipe

A FLAVOR FOR ALL SEASONS

BEAUTIFYING GOMASIO

Seasoning your meal can multiply its beauty benefits, especially if you look to global traditions. Take gomasio, a mineral-rich, time-honored condiment with Japanese origins. Gomasio is delicious when added to warm veggies or grain bowls after cooking, or atop avocado toast. You may even use it as a nutrient-packed replacement for salt and pepper. The sesame seeds in the mix are full of zinc and healthy fats, while dulse seaweed adds metabolism-supporting iodine and B_6 and protein for gorgeous hair.

MAKES ABOUT ⅓ CUP [47 G]

5 Tbsp [40 g] sesame seeds (golden, white, or black)
1 Tbsp dulse flakes

¼ tsp ground cumin
⅛ tsp unrefined salt

In a small skillet over medium heat, gently toast the sesame seeds, stirring constantly, until lightly browned and fragrant, about 2 minutes. Immediately transfer the seeds to a bowl to prevent scorching. Stir in the dulse, cumin, and salt and crush the mixture with the back of the spoon, gently grinding the ingredients together. Transfer to a shaker bottle or airtight container and store in the refrigerator for up to six months.

Kitchen Inspiration

❧ COCONUT PRODUCTS ❧

These days, coconut can be purchased in so many different forms—coconut water, coconut oil, coconut flour, and coconut sugar, to name a few—that it can be overwhelming to know which offer the most beauty benefits. The answer depends on your diet and preferences, but I have a few favorites: coconut oil, coconut milk, and coconut butter, as well as unsweetened coconut flakes, from which coconut butter is ground. Because these particular products are made or extracted from whole, fresh coconuts, they deliver anti-inflammatory medium-chain fats (which are excellent for energy and metabolism) as well as the antimicrobial fat lauric acid—what I see as the two most beneficial nutritional components of coconuts. As for other coconut products, they don't include as many of the beauty-supporting fats, but they do have their own distinct benefits. For example, coconut water is excellent for quick rehydration and electrolyte balance, making it a great post-workout thirst quencher. Coconut flour is an iron- and fiber-rich, gluten-free flour, while coconut sugar is a low glycemic sugar alternative made from the sap of the palm tree. Swap them into a dessert recipe when you want to make a skin-friendly treat.

Time for Self-Love

❧ RELAX INTO ACUPUNCTURE ❧

Next time you're in need of some serious self-love and rejuvenation, schedule an acupuncture session. You may already be a devotee, or you may be thinking, "Wait—sticking needles in my skin is a form of pampering?" It totally is, and more. But don't just take it from me—experience it for yourself. Some of the benefits of acupuncture (which aims to balance the flow of energy, or *qi*, throughout the body with the strategic placement of fine, hair-width needles) are increased energy, a feeling of positivity or calm, release of emotion, and even relief of built-up pain and tension. When something's out of balance with your body—which inevitably affects your beauty—but you just can't pinpoint exactly what you need, acupuncture is an ideal therapy to try. It's another form of listening to your body's needs and responding in a beautifying way. And, if wrinkles are on your radar, there's a specific form of acupuncture, called cosmetic acupuncture, that aims to increase collagen production to counteract skin wrinkling.

Beauty Science
NOTICE HAIR AND NAILS

Are you seeing less-than-lustrous hair in the mirror, or noticing slow-to-grow nails? When your diet is lacking in nutrients, your hair and nails are some of the first places to show a deficiency—a result of a slowdown in your body's production of keratin, a key protein they share. One study found that supplementing your diet with a combination of vitamins A, C, E, and B complex, plus minerals zinc, magnesium, and iron (an array that you'll find in a good multivitamin, or a well-rounded beauty diet) significantly boosted keratin production.

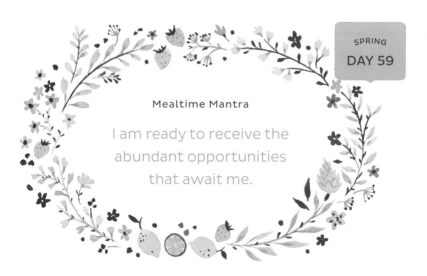

Mealtime Mantra

I am ready to receive the abundant opportunities that await me.

Intention of the Week
❧ RETRAIN YOUR BREATHING ❧

Of course you know how to breathe. But do you know how to breathe for beauty? Doing so can trigger your parasympathetic nervous system and produce a calming effect throughout the body. Each day this week, try this simple technique: Breathe deeply and slowly in through your nose, letting your lower abdomen expand instead of your chest. Exhale naturally, but slightly longer than your inhale. When you've mastered this simple yet challenging technique and enter a relaxed breath rhythm, try to extend it for ten minutes a day—while at your desk, driving, walking, or wherever you might otherwise be breathing quick, shallow breaths. You'll support waste removal through your deep exhalations, and activate a calming response that supports hormone balance and healthy aging.

Time for Self-Love

WALK AND MEDITATE

If you want to experience the calming, mind-focusing benefits of meditation but can't seem to settle your restless body into a sitting session, walking meditation could be a good fit for you. If you've ever lost yourself in a meditative state during a long walk, you know that it's an effective way to shut out your to-do list and deeply relax both your mind and your body. To practice walking meditation, find a place to walk outdoors, in a park, around a lake, on a path through woods or forest, or even down a city street (perhaps the most challenging option, given the ample distractions). Take a slow, relaxed walk while you breathe deeply and focus on the sensations you experience: the way your feet feel as they hit the ground, the effect of the breeze hitting your face, the sunlight in your eyes, or your arms swinging. If thoughts other than those about the act of walking enter your mind, let them go, just as you would during sitting meditation. Reduced stress, greater mindfulness and calm, and digestive support are just some of the beauty benefits of a regular meditation practice.

Living Your Best Life

HOW TO DETOX YOUR DEODORANT

One of your body's key detox mechanisms is sweating. To support this healthy process, and protect the sensitive underarm area near your breasts, make sure your deodorant contains ingredients that counteract odor without bringing along potentially toxic compounds like aluminum, synthetic fragrance, or paraben preservatives. When choosing a natural deodorant, look for active ingredients like cornstarch, activated charcoal, baking soda, coconut oil, natural clays, and essential oils. You might consider asking your friends if they've found an effective natural deodorant—but note that deodorant formulas work better on some bodies than others, so your friend's must-have product may not be the one for you. When you make the switch, you may notice that it takes your body a week or two to adjust; give it time and try a few formulas until you find the perfect match. The effort is worth it for your body's long-term health!

Kitchen Inspiration
HAIR SUPERFOODS

Is your hair looking dull, flat, or weak? Rather than turning to yet another hair product, see what beauty nutrition can do for you. Strengthening your hair from the inside out can be even more impactful in the long run than hair products. To boost hair health over time, first be sure you're getting enough easily digestible protein, which is the building block of keratin (and in turn, healthy hair). About 45 g a day is the protein intake recommendation for an average woman, but that varies individually, so ask your doctor what amount is right for you. Wild salmon, hemp seeds, quinoa, sardines, and plant-based protein powders are a few of the best protein choices for beauty. Additionally, opt for foods rich in hair-building minerals like iron and zinc, for example raw pumpkin seeds, oysters, leafy greens, and lentils, as well as elasticity-supporting silicon, found in bananas, gluten-free oats, and radishes. Finally, support optimal digestion of these nutrients with a daily probiotic supplement or fermented foods like miso and kimchi.

Time for Self-Love

PREVENT SNACK ATTACKS

If you reach for sweets, coffee, or a bag of chips each afternoon, chances are you haven't filled up on enough nutritious foods during the earlier part of your day. Give yourself permission to add more whole, unprocessed vegetables and fruits, clean proteins, and healthy fats to your breakfast and lunch—especially if you're regularly feeling afternoon hunger and fatigue. When you eat a satisfying breakfast and lunch, afternoon junk food loses its luster. Of course, if you're eating satisfying meals and *still* getting afternoon cravings, start packing a beautifying snack and indulge the healthy way.

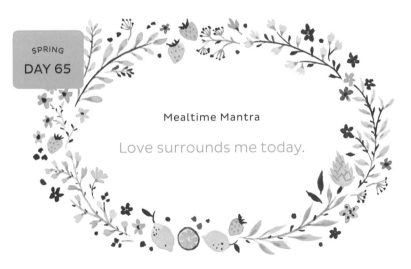

Mealtime Mantra

Love surrounds me today.

Intention of the Week

LOWER WRINKLE-PROMOTING AGEs IN YOUR DIET

AGEs, or advanced glycation end products, are compounds that form rigid bonds in the proteins in your skin (as well as in your muscles and bones), contributing to wrinkling, sagging, and thinning. Higher AGE levels mean more inflammation and additional free radicals in the body, creating an all-around tough situation for beauty. Some of the biggest contributors to AGEs in the body come from our diet—specifically sugar, refined carbs, processed foods, burned or overcooked foods, and foods (especially meats) that are cooked with high, dry heat methods like roasting, broiling, and grilling. This week, take action to reduce the AGEs in your diet with these scientifically proven methods: Build your diet around vegetables, legumes, fish, fruit, and whole grains, and use low AGE–forming cooking methods like steaming, boiling, poaching, and quick, low-heat cooking. Using acidic marinades like vinegar and lemon juice can lower AGE formation on grilled foods. Some examples of beautifying meals that are low in AGEs are a vegetable-packed seafood stew or a quinoa bowl with steamed vegetables and beans. Try to create your own low-AGE meals this week, and incorporate them into your diet whenever you can to reduce your overall AGE intake.

Beauty Food Profile
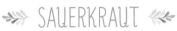
SAUERKRAUT

Get your hands on kraut—the kind you ferment at home (see the recipe on page 113) or find in the refrigerated section of your grocery store labeled "raw," "fermented," and/or "live"—for the digestive beauty benefits you've been missing! A healthy digestive system is closely connected to radiant skin, immunity, good moods, and a healthy weight, making pungent sauerkraut an unexpected beauty food. Sauerkraut that's been fermented is a concentrated source of beneficial bacteria for your body, so much so that a few forkfuls can far surpass the benefits of a probiotic supplement. Sauerkraut that's made from cabbage has an excellent dose of highly absorbable collagen-building vitamin C; vitamins K_1 and K_2 for healthy blood vessels, bones, and teeth; and iron. You will also see krauts made with other fermented veggies; these will have a slightly different nutritional profile, but just as many probiotic benefits. Try adding a small serving of sauerkraut to your diet each day to improve your digestion and see a positive difference in your skin.

EAT PRETTY FOOD	BEAUTIFYING COMPOUND	BEAUTY BENEFIT
Sauerkraut	Beneficial bacteria	Support digestive health and elimination

Beauty Science

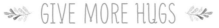

GIVE MORE HUGS

A feeling of happiness benefits both beauty and health, but how do we get more of that in our day-to-day life? One science-backed way to surge the happiness-building brain chemical oxytocin is to tap into the power of touch. Hold or shake hands. Get a massage. Cuddle a loved one. And give hugs! One study found that participants who gave or received a minimum of five hugs a day for one week reported a significant boost in happiness. Hugging (the longer the better) also lowers the stress hormone cortisol, further supporting optimal beauty.

Time for Self-Love
DISCOVER YOUR
WORKOUT SWEET SPOT

You've heard study after study praising the health benefits of regular exercise. While exercise *is* a healthy beauty
essential, the whole truth is that exercise, like diet, isn't
one size fits all. Some workouts can negatively impact
your hormone balance, even as you're pushing yourself
to work harder, run faster, and come away stronger. Here
are a few clues to watch for, indicating that your workout
may not be right for you right now: you feel drained after
exercise instead of energized with a good-mood endorphin boost; you're working out hard but the scale won't
budge; you dread your workout like you dread doing your
taxes. If this is you, switch things up. Many women find
that an intense sweat session plus an intense day at the
office throws their stress hormone cortisol into overdrive,
resulting in breakouts, redness, and stubborn weight that
just won't come off. If this sounds familiar, balance your
energetic workouts with walking, yoga, strength train-
ing, and stretching and breathing, and see if it's a better
fit. Keep in mind that your body's needs are frequently
shifting. The workout that suits you best today may
change again next week—it's up to you to listen to your
body and to remember that you *don't* always need pain
to gain beauty and balance.

Kitchen Inspiration

A GREEN BEAUTY BOOSTER

One of my favorite go-to green boosters for energy, immunity, and beauty benefits between meals are chlorella tabs, made from broken-down chlorella, a nutrient-rich algae. Chlorella is packed with beta-carotene, chlorophyll, iron, and B vitamins, beauty nutrients that also reduce aging levels of oxidative stress. Since the tabs digest easily, they can be swallowed whole. Chase them with a glass of water for a hydration boost. For best results, look for high-quality chlorella that's been tested to be free of heavy metals.

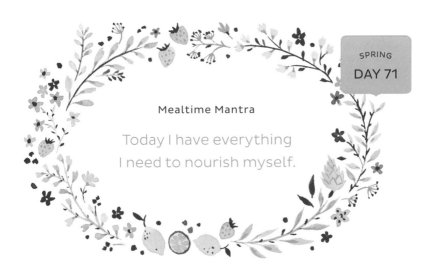

Mealtime Mantra

Today I have everything
I need to nourish myself.

Intention of the Week

WORK ON REDUCING STRESS EACH DAY

There are all too many looming stressors in our lives, whether from work, home life, a hectic commute, or a never-ending to-do list. Managing that stress and teaching our bodies to reduce, or turn off, our stress response is one of the most powerful things we can do for our lifelong beauty. Studies show that high levels of the stress hormone cortisol result in collagen loss in the skin at a far greater rate than in other tissues. Cortisol also creates inflammation in the body, making it harder to achieve a healthy weight and balanced hormones. As you go about your daily routine in the week ahead, look for opportunities to reduce stress and prevent the release of cortisol in your body. Here are a few tried-and-true methods: spend time in nature, seek out good company, meditate, laugh, move, eat more vitamin C, and breathe deeply. Do more of the things that make you feel happy and worry free, even for a moment.

Eat Pretty Recipe

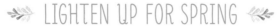

LIGHTEN UP FOR SPRING

WARMING SPRING SOUP

Spring is the season to fill your plate—or bowl—with light, detoxifying beauty foods, many of them raw. But on days when an unexpected cold snap hits, your body will crave the cozy warmth of cooked foods. This recipe gathers some of spring's freshest, most detox-friendly green beauty foods into a light, nourishing soup that chases away a chill.

SERVES 4 TO 6

1 tsp coconut oil

4 shallots, chopped

10 oz [280 g] white button or cremini mushrooms, brushed clean and chopped

4 oz [115 g] shiitake mushroom caps, brushed clean and chopped

2 cloves garlic, minced

1 Tbsp fresh thyme leaves

8 cups [2 L] vegetable broth

1½ cups [170 g] gluten-free rotini pasta

1 cup [140 g] fresh or frozen peas

2 large handfuls fresh organic spinach, chopped

Unrefined salt and freshly ground black pepper

In a large pot, melt the coconut oil over medium heat. Add the shallots and cook until they begin to soften. Add the mushrooms, garlic, and thyme and cook until the mushrooms are tender and reduced, 5 to 8 minutes. Add the broth and raise the heat to high. When the broth begins to steam, add the pasta. Simmer for about 10 minutes, stirring once or twice to prevent the pasta from sticking. Stir in the peas and spinach and cook until the spinach wilts and the pasta is just tender, about 5 minutes longer. Season with salt and pepper. Ladle into bowls and serve immediately.

Living Your Best Life
HOW TO RESET YOUR BODY

When your digestion feels off, your skin looks upset, your cravings are out of control, or you've gone a bit too far off track with your diet, it could be time to reset your body. For a truly beautifying way to bring your body back into balance without complicated rules and restrictions, all you may need to do is think of how you can simplify your diet. This might mean reducing the number of add-ins, additives, and options you fill your plate with—for just one meal, one day, or a few weeks. It might also mean making a nourishing soup, a smoothie, or a simple stir-fry using just a few ingredients. Or it might mean eating smaller portions for a day (or three). These simple strategies give your body a chance to recharge and reset. This spring, listen to your body and reset it with gentleness.

Kitchen Inspiration

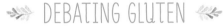
DEBATING GLUTEN

Some say gluten-free eating is merely a fad, while others insist that every person on the planet should shun gluten for life. I don't believe in either of those extremes. But depending on your individual body, as well as where you live on the globe, gluten could be a catalyst for some significant beauty issues in your body, so it's important to be aware of how it affects you personally. Gluten can cause inflammation, water retention, and bloating, and the nature of many gluten-containing foods is neither nutrient-dense nor beauty-friendly. But the same can be said for many gluten-free processed foods, so it's hard to point a finger at gluten alone! All things considered, should you keep your kitchen gluten free? Strictly for beauty and skin health, my vote is yes, but you have to make the call for yourself. If you're interested in exploring the gluten-free lifestyle, try a period of time without gluten in your diet, or your kitchen, to understand how it's affecting you; and to support the process, pack your meals with whole foods that are naturally gluten-free, like a rainbow of produce, healthy fats like raw nuts and avocado, and clean proteins like wild salmon and quinoa.

Pretty Pairing

PASTURED EGGS + ORGANIC COLLARD GREENS

Why they're more beautiful together: Next time you make an omelet, sauté up some chopped, organic collard greens to stuff inside. The vitamin D content of pastured eggs helps the body absorb the beautifying dose of calcium that collard greens provide, while also calming nervous function, assisting with skin cell production, and maintaining strong bones and teeth.

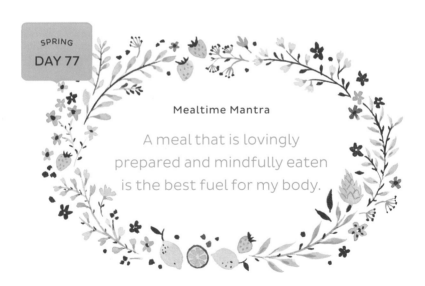

Mealtime Mantra

A meal that is lovingly prepared and mindfully eaten is the best fuel for my body.

Time for Self-Love

CREATE MOMENTS FOR BEAUTY

You know those repetitive tasks that you perform again and again, like washing your face? Make an effort to turn them into moments for beauty. We often forget that small indulgences can have the most beautifying impact in our day-to-day routine. For example, to turn face-washing into a moment you'll look forward to, buy a stack of organic cotton washcloths. (Splurge on the super-soft, super-luxurious kind!) After cleansing and rinsing, dampen a washcloth with warm water and use it to perform a gentle, final rinse. In doing so, you'll more thoroughly remove cleanser residue and introduce extra exfoliation that keeps skin smooth and even, thus allowing your post-washing products to penetrate better. Pamper yourself by using a fresh washcloth each time you cleanse.

Intention of the Week

EAT MORE RAW FOODS

Cold, crunchy veggies on a bone-chilling winter evening might not sound very satisfying. But in springtime, as the days get longer, the sun gets stronger, and your body and beauty enter a natural detox phase, you'll find raw foods to be the perfect addition to your plate. Among other benefits, they're packed with naturally occurring enzymes that help you digest and assimilate their nutrition optimally and cleanse other toxins from the body. Raw foods (which technically can be lightly cooked, as long as they're not heated to a temperature over 116°F [47°C]) cleanse the lymphatic system, which supports radiant skin and reduced cellulite, and can provide a powerful alkaline boost for the body. This week, savor a salad, dive into a vibrant plate of crudités, or blend up a raw soup that will cleanse and refresh your palate and your beauty, inside and out.

Beauty Food Profile

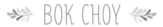 BOK CHOY

Bok choy is a cruciferous vegetable related to the cabbage that's growing in demand, in part due to its powerful anti-aging nutrition. Characterized by its pretty, sweet, and crunchy pure-white stalks and leafy green tops, bok choy is among the top-ranked veggies for nutrient density, and is also being studied for its cancer-preventive properties. It scores high for collagen-boosting vitamin C, beta-carotene (which converts to skin-smoothing, healing vitamin A), calcium, and potassium. Bok choy contains a range of phytochemicals that defend against aging, including lutein and zeaxanthin for eye health, indole-3-carbinol for hormone balance, and sulforaphane for a boost in glutathione and a reduction in redness after UV exposure. Add big or baby bok choy to a stir-fry or soup for extra crunch and a new level of anti-aging nutrition.

EAT PRETTY FOOD	BEAUTIFYING COMPOUND	BEAUTY BENEFIT
Bok choy	Sulforaphane	Boosts glutathione production

Living Your Best Life

HOW TO INCLUDE RESISTANT STARCH IN YOUR DIET

Just like calories, not all carbs are created equal. And an overwhelming amount of research shows that one particular type of carb, called "resistant starch," has the power to lower your blood sugar levels (remember, spiking blood sugar has links to blemishes, wrinkles, and weight gain), boost fat burning, benefit digestion, and keep you feeling fuller. Resistant starch is aptly named, as it resists digestion in your stomach and small intestine—meaning you don't absorb as many calories from foods in the resistant starch category. Also beneficial to beauty, resistant starches feed good bacteria in our digestive systems that produce a particular fatty acid called butyrate, which supports fat burning, lowered inflammation, and colon health. To get more healthy resistant starch in your diet, munch on corn, raw nuts and seeds, plantains and slightly underripe bananas, cooked and cooled rice, quinoa, and other grains, as well as cooked and cooled sweet potatoes, white potatoes, and beans.

Time for Self-Love

MAKE ROOM FOR ENERGIZING RELATIONSHIPS

This spring, the season of shedding and lightening, consider the relationships, romantic or otherwise, that drain you or leave you feeling negative or regretful. While social connection is vital for stress relief and a balanced life, some relationships have a greater number of healthy benefits than others. Prioritize the connections that fulfill you, and let the others fall away. Use the extra room in your schedule, or in your social media circle, to open yourself up to new relationships that may bring fresh doses of positive energy into your life.

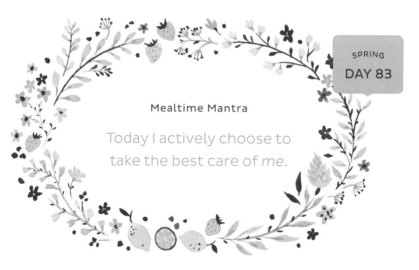

Mealtime Mantra

Today I actively choose to take the best care of *me*.

Kitchen Inspiration

LIVER-SUPPORTING NUTRITION

Your liver, a major source of waste filtering and total-body detoxification, is an important organ to keep in top shape if radiant skin is your goal. You can help lighten the daily load on your liver by supporting healthy digestion and elimination and skipping as many of the Beauty Betrayers (foods like alcohol, conventional meats and dairy, processed foods, and sugars that tax your beauty and body—see page 10) as you can. There are also quite a few foods that help your liver stay at the peak of its health and detoxifying abilities. Include these liver-loving vegetables and fruits in your beauty diet regularly to nourish radiant skin: apples, artichokes, asparagus, beets, burdock root, cabbage, dandelion and other leafy greens, lemons, limes, parsley, and sprouts.

Intention of the Week

HAVE FUN MOVING FOR THIRTY MINUTES EACH DAY

Finding different forms of exercise that you enjoy is key to maintaining this beautifying habit for life. Research shows that physical activity that makes you happy has even more profound health benefits than the physical activity you do while completing chores that you don't like, or slogging through exercise that feels like work. Walking or doing other exercise for pleasure appears to have the biggest positive impact on mental well-being, mood, and longevity. Personal experience may tell you this is true, too. This week, opt for physical activity that doesn't feel like a task. Try to enjoy it for at least thirty minutes every day. If you're stuck for ideas, take a walk with a friend—or perhaps offer to babysit a child you love and have them show you their favorite sport!

Beauty Food Profile

NUTRITIONAL YEAST

We hear a lot about yeasts that are problematic for the body, but there are a few yeasts that are quite beneficial. Nutritional yeast and brewer's yeast are two that are full of healthy benefits. The difference in their names is meant to distinguish whether the yeast was grown during the beer-making process (brewer's yeast), or on other foods like beets (nutritional yeast). All you really need to know is that these yeasts are powerhouse sources of B vitamins, protein, and beauty minerals like iron and zinc. They make an excellent food-based supplement for B vitamins, which support our skin, hair and nails, nervous system, and energy level. Some studies have linked brewer's yeast to acne improvement; however, it's important to pay close attention to your own reaction to yeast supplementation and make sure it benefits you. Some people love these yeasts for their "cheesy" taste as well, and will use them in any situation that calls for grated Parmesan—if you want to try this substitution, try different brands, as they have very different flavors and you'll need to find the one you like best. You can sprinkle it on popcorn, chili, salads, scrambled eggs, and other savory dishes, or use it to boost the flavor and beauty benefits of sauces and dressings.

EAT PRETTY FOOD	BEAUTIFYING COMPOUND	BEAUTY BENEFIT
Nutritional yeast	B-complex vitamins	Nourish skin, hair, and nails

Beauty Science

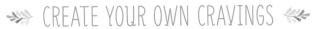 CREATE YOUR OWN CRAVINGS

Skeptical that you could ever become addicted to watercress? According to one study, you can! The study showed that, in just six months' time, your brain can boost the reward signals that it releases when you eat healthy foods and decrease its addiction to unhealthy foods. So, start incorporating beauty foods into your diet today and by the fall you (or your brain) will be hooked.

My top pick for beauty foods to get hooked on this spring are bitter and peppery greens like dandelion, arugula, and watercress, which are fabulous detoxifiers filled with the skin-repairing nutrition your body needs after a long winter. Develop your tastes for these strong, beautifying greens and you'll eat your way to a more youthful complexion in a few short weeks.

Kitchen Inspiration
ELIMINATE ENDOCRINE DISRUPTORS

Many canned goods are lined with a protective inner coating that contains bisphenol A (BPA), an endocrine-disrupting chemical that is also found in plastics and printed store receipts. BPA has been linked to breast cancer and hormonal issues. Do some research into the brands of canned goods that you buy and make sure you choose those that are BPA free. While you're at it, phase out your plastic storage and microwave containers and replace them with durable, long-lasting glass containers that won't release endocrine-disrupting chemicals when heated or when they get worn out.

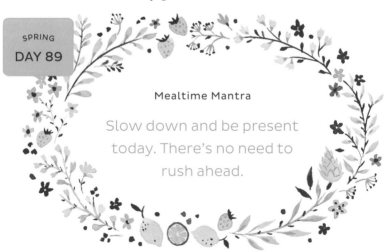

Mealtime Mantra

Slow down and be present today. There's no need to rush ahead.

Beauty Food Profile

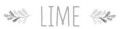 LIME

If you love the beauty benefits of your morning lemon water but want to experiment with a different flavor profile, bring limes into your kitchen. Like lemons, limes are powerful liver detoxifiers, highly alkaline, and loaded with antioxidant vitamin C (about a quarter of your daily needs are in the juice of one lime). Limes are slightly sweeter and less acidic than lemons, and still incredibly low in sugar and calories. Use them in smoothies and dressings just as you would use lemons.

EAT PRETTY FOOD	BEAUTIFYING COMPOUND	BEAUTY BENEFIT
Lime	Vitamin C	Powerful antioxidant defender

Intention of the Week

PLAN AN AFTERNOON PICK-ME-UP

Often our afternoon rituals (you know, the ones that provide instant gratification but sabotage skin and energy, like a late-afternoon coffee run or a trip to the office vending machine for a candy pick-me-up) can feel like they're good for us because of the surge of energy they provide. This makes it easy to rationalize what is actually just a junk-food fix. This week, spend some time dreaming up an afternoon ritual that you'll look forward to even more than caffeine or sugar—one that boosts your beauty instead of working against it. My top picks are an afternoon stretching session (or a mini nap, if you can swing it), a walk around the block alone or with a friend or colleague, or taking a few minutes to prepare a skin-friendly smoothie or fruit-infused water. You'll find that a little bit of self-care transforms your mood and energy—and satisfies your body's cravings in an unexpected way.

≫ GOODBYE, SPRING. HELLO, SUMMER! ≪

Having read more than ninety Eat Pretty tips during this season, you should feel refreshed and ready to jump into the energy and heat of summer. As you do so, retain your spring-inspired practices and know that they will support you in any season. Start off your days with a positive outlook, lemon water, and a beauty-fueling breakfast. Eat an abundance of greens, embrace beautifying new habits, reduce your exposure to toxic products, and, in general, fill your plate with fresh, whole, and lightly cooked foods. The ability to balance your body by shifting your meals and habits with the seasons is an intuitive skill you'll develop even more in the seasons to come. Tomorrow, a new season awaits, filled with a fresh crop of ideas to nourish your beauty through the sun-filled summertime. Each summer day brings new opportunities to care for your beauty and body, and a new page of inspiration to guide you ahead toward your best self. Turn the page and create your summer glow.

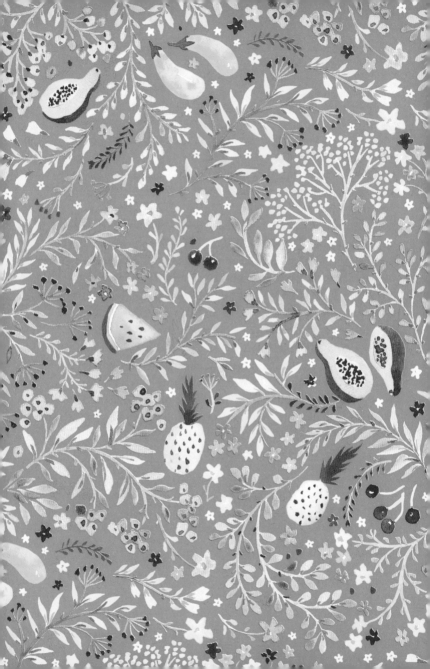

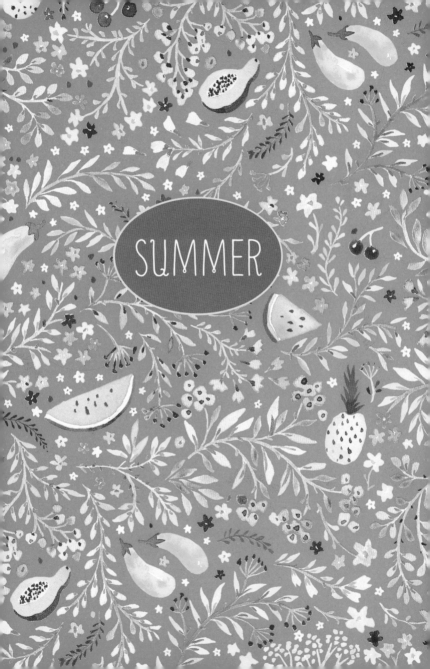

SUMMER

Summer is the season of the sun, a source of life and light that reflects your own radiating energy and beauty. Embrace daily opportunities to move, play, connect with nature, and enjoy the colorful variety of beauty foods available to you this season. At the same time, honor your need to relax and recharge at intervals too, since summer brings with it extremes in temperatures and activity that can throw you and your beauty into a tailspin. Each entry in the pages ahead encourages you to find that ideal balance.

This season, you'll learn to build beauty by bringing more joy and self-love into your life, along with an abundance of nature's best summer beauty foods. Ahead, you'll find more than ninety entries to guide you. You'll seek out activities that let you move, laugh, sweat, and strengthen your body. You'll soak up the outdoors, and balance the aging effects of increased sun exposure with sun protection from natural ingredients and sun-protective foods like watermelon, tomatoes, wild salmon, and red peppers. You'll eat seasonally from the plant-based spectrum of colors and flavors you have available to you in the summer, and hydrate your body with plenty of pure water and water-rich summer foods like cucumber, zucchini, and peaches. And you'll fuel yourself with clean proteins like wild salmon, quinoa, lentils, and pastured eggs that stabilize your blood sugar and give you lasting energy to savor longer days. Look for new ideas in these pages that could become regular habits in your lifestyle of beauty. Find practices for your life that make you feel passionate. What truly lights your fire this season?

As summer days pass, don't forget to look in the mirror and love the incredible glow that you have going on. Be a light for others, showing them how profoundly they can influence the appearance of their own skin, hair, nails, weight, energy, and moods with a few small changes to their diet and lifestyle. Turn the page, read the first entry, and make it your most beautiful summer yet.

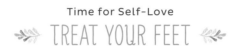

Time for Self-Love

TREAT YOUR FEET

Our underappreciated feet take a real beating over the course of an average day, and we tend not to blink an eye at blisters, soreness, or swelling and stiffness in our toes, heels, and soles. To show your feet some extra care and feel whole-body benefits, try foot massage, a gratifying and underutilized self-care ritual. According to the teachings of reflexology, there are thousands of extremely sensitive nerve endings in our feet that, when stimulated by touch, affect our overall health and beauty in dramatic ways. Regardless of whether or not you can actually improve your digestion by touching the center sole of your foot (one of the point-to-point connections made in reflexology), simple foot massage can stimulate circulation and the nervous system, soften feet, and deeply relax the body. Keep your favorite cream or body oil at your bedside and massage your clean, dry soles in circular motions with your thumbs, in one direction and then the other, before you crawl into bed. You'll certainly calm your mind, and your feet just may look more beautiful when you slip on heels or sandals again the next day.

Kitchen Inspiration

A FRESH ALTERNATIVE TO THE SUMMER BBQ

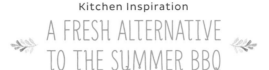

Summer's go-to gathering may be a barbecue, but there's more than one skin-supportive reason to step out from behind the hot grill. Grilled foods, especially those that have been browned or charred over high heat, contain high amounts of wrinkle-forming AGEs (advanced glycation end products). Make your next summer gathering festive and seasonal by serving a dish—or an entire meal—that features raw instead of grilled ingredients. Instead of charring asparagus spears, serve them raw with a homemade dressing for dipping (page 61). In place of a grilled protein, serve a chilled quinoa salad, which also has the benefits of complete protein. Your guests will love the keep-cool, no-grill theme—especially when they learn about the bonus beautifying nutrients and digestive enzymes in your cool, crunchy and ultra-fresh summer food.

Living Your Best Life

HOW TO LOOK AND FEEL YOUR BEST WHILE TRAVELING

To arrive at your far-off destination feeling great, beautify while you travel. In addition to the requisite refillable water bottle and stack of magazines you'll pack in your carry-on, assemble a few key items for beauty and wellness before your next flight. At the top of my list are 1) a meditation or relaxation app that will help me relax in flight or calm any anxieties that crop up while I'm away from home; 2) aromatherapy oils (try a roll-on oil blend with lavender or neroli for their well-documented calming properties); 3) a hydrating facial toner to spray over my face and neck several times during the skin-drying journey; and 4) supplements such as digestive enzymes and probiotics to keep digestion regular on the road. It's these little things that maintain your body and beauty balance, no matter where your summer trip takes you!

Intention of the Week

ADD MORE BEAUTIFYING FIBER TO YOUR DIET

Here's a delicious beauty secret: one super-simple way to support your healthiest weight is to boost your fiber intake. Eating about 30 g of fiber each day can improve both weight loss and insulin resistance—a measure of how well the body responds to insulin, which is an important factor in aging. That's the result of an increase in fiber intake *alone*; no other diet or lifestyle changes involved! Another benefit of fiber is its ability to support natural detox, hormone balance, and microbial diversity in your gut. So what's the easiest way to increase your fiber (and add additional beauty benefits to your diet while you're at it)? Think seeds: chia, hemp, flax, and sunflower; berries with seeds count too. Sprinkle these into your smoothie or atop your salad to get all the benefits fiber has to offer. Other fiber-rich beauty foods include chickpeas, kidney beans, broccoli, and quinoa. Remember: getting your fiber from whole, plant-based foods has even more beauty benefits than a fiber supplement.

Beauty Science

❦ TAKE TIME TO SMELL THE ROSES ❦

Research suggests that the scent of roses has a multitude of beauty benefits. One study found that inhaling rose essential oil reduces several negative effects: the skin's inflammatory response to stress (which can cause redness and breakouts); levels of the stress hormone cortisol; and the skin's water loss, keeping it better hydrated. Another study found that smelling fresh roses activates the body's relaxing parasympathetic nervous system. Add some rose essential oil to your diffuser or order yourself a bouquet of summer roses the next time your skin and mind need calming!

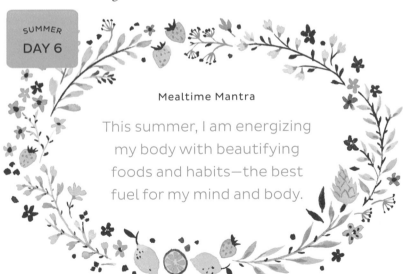

Mealtime Mantra

This summer, I am energizing my body with beautifying foods and habits—the best fuel for my mind and body.

Beauty Food Profile

BLACKBERRIES

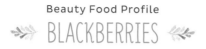

These dark, juicy jewels are brimming with anti-inflammatory, antioxidant phytochemicals, including anthocyanins, known for their ability to support skin elasticity and brain health and defend against DNA damage, and ellagic acid, which aids in blood sugar balance and defends against skin wrinkling. Blackberries and their fibrous seeds are excellent for digestive health, and contain collagen-building vitamin C as well as the beauty minerals iron and manganese for gorgeous hair and mitochondrial function. Blackberries also happen to be one of the few alkaline fruits, making them especially supportive of healthy pH balance in the body.

EAT PRETTY FOOD	BEAUTIFYING COMPOUND	BEAUTY BENEFIT
Blackberries	Anthocyanins	Support skin elasticity

Time for Self-Love

STRAIGHTEN UP

You already know that changing your posture can make you look taller, but does the way you hold your body have the power to influence beauty on a deeper level? You bet. In recent studies, standing or sitting upright—spine straight, shoulders back—corresponded with lower levels of the stress hormone cortisol; feelings of enthusiasm, excitement, and strength; improved confidence and self-esteem; and even a stronger pulse. Plus, good posture allows for deeper, more complete breaths and therefore increased oxygen, an essential for circulation and waste removal in the body. Stand tall, and you experience an instant mind-body beauty boost.

Eat Pretty Recipe

DIY PROBIOTICS

GINGERED PURPLE KRAUT

Eating fermented foods daily is my favorite way to nourish a healthy gut, which supports radiant skin, a healthy weight, resilience to stress, and fewer allergies. You can find premade krauts at the grocery store, or you can ferment at home—it's easier than you think!

MAKES A 1-QUART JAR OF KRAUT

1 head red cabbage, about 2 lb [910 g], cored and very thinly sliced, 1 or 2 large outer leaves reserved	2-in [5-cm] knob of fresh ginger, peeled and finely grated 4 tsp unrefined salt

In a large bowl, combine the shredded cabbage, ginger, and salt. Using clean hands, toss to mix well. Let sit for 20 minutes, periodically squeezing the cabbage mixture to release moisture. When the cabbage feels wilted and brine has collected in the bowl, squeeze well once more. Tightly pack the cabbage mixture into a clean 1-qt [960-ml] jar. When you reach the shoulders of the jar, stop filling.

Fold and stuff the reserved cabbage leaves into the jar, pressing down firmly. Weigh down the leaves with a smaller jar, sterilized stone, or other clean, heavy object and pour in the brine remaining in the bowl until all of the cabbage is under liquid. Cover with a clean kitchen towel and secure the towel tightly with a rubber band around the neck. Let your kraut ferment at room temperature until it reaches your desired flavor, 2 to 3 weeks, then transfer to the fridge; it's ready to consume!

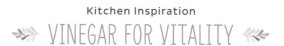

Kitchen Inspiration

VINEGAR FOR VITALITY

The act of drinking vinegar may sound like a middle-school dare, but in fact it can be a beautifying practice at any age. Apple cider vinegar (look for the raw, fermented kind) is a strongly alkaline food that helps to balance the pH of your body as well as lower inflammation and support healthy digestion, as it contains beneficial bacteria and increases the acidity of the stomach. Consuming apple cider vinegar also lowers blood-sugar levels (its acetic acid slows the digestion of carbs), making it a great tool for healthy aging and youthful skin. If you're not keen on sipping it undiluted, add water and sometimes lemon or honey, or both, for a soothing beauty tonic, or splash in sparkling water for a fizzy, flavorful sip. I like to add it to homemade dressings to enjoy its beautifying benefits in a salad.

Time for Self-Love
HONOR YOUR COMMITMENT TO YOURSELF

Find a token—such as a charm hanging on a simple chain, a pretty gemstone, or a string of mala beads traditionally used for meditation—and let it symbolize your commitment and intention to honor your lifelong beauty and health. Make sure it feels like a true expression of your own unique beauty and energy. This physical item is something that you can look to again and again for inspiration and as a reminder to weave self-love and healthy vanity into every day of your beautiful life.

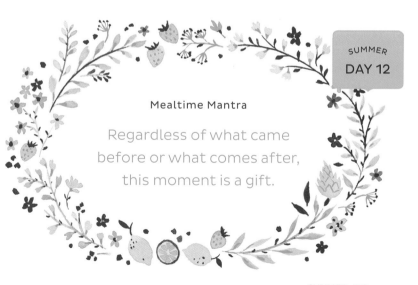

Mealtime Mantra

Regardless of what came before or what comes after, this moment is a gift.

Intention of the Week

SPEND MORE TIME OUTDOORS

Don't overlook a beauty booster that's available to you at no cost, in rain or shine: time spent outdoors. The hours we spend inside—at our computers, traveling around in cars, buses, and trains, always in heated or air conditioned climates—vastly outnumber the hours we spend seeing, breathing, and staying in touch with the natural world around us. It's become the norm to miss out on the scientifically proven stress-lowering effects of time spent in nature, whether that nature is a city park or a quiet meadow. Seize opportunities to get outdoors each day this week, and your stress-induced, age-advancing cortisol levels will plummet, even as your pleasure and perspective grow.

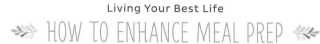

Living Your Best Life

HOW TO ENHANCE MEAL PREP

Kitchen gadgets and tools can overhaul the way you cook and multiply your options for preparing meals from whole, fresh ingredients—not to mention make meal prep more fun. I think the most useful kitchen tool—beyond knives, pots, and pans, of course—is a blender or food processor. These high-powered machines will transform the way you make smoothies, soups, dips, nut butters, flours, and raw desserts. Another game-changing tool is a simple mandoline, a manual wonder that allows you to slice veggies quickly and uniformly. Lastly, a spinner for drying your greens will get endless use in a home where greens are a staple. In addition to these three tools, you might find that there's a particular gadget that suits your unique preferences and simply makes your meals happier—perhaps an avocado slicer, which does the job in just one neat chop, or a spiralizer, which makes pastalike noodles from vegetables like zucchini and beets. Fill your kitchen with the tools that make your meals feel joyful as well as convenient, and those that inspire your creative process.

Kitchen Inspiration

COLORFUL RICE

You probably have white and brown rice in your pantry, but consider adding black rice (sometimes called purple or "longevity rice") to the mix to enjoy its unique beauty benefits. The dark bran of the black rice kernel contains anthocyanins (similar to what's found in the skins of blueberries and plums), which are known to provide antioxidants, protect DNA, and boost skin elasticity. One study found that ten spoonfuls of cooked black rice has about the same dose of anthocyanins as one spoonful of blueberries, making the rice a well-kept secret source of extra beauty nutrition for your skin. Black rice takes longer to cook (unless you soak it beforehand), but you can sub it for brown rice in all kinds of recipes. For extra nutritional benefits and unique flavor, try cooking it in broth or tea.

Time for Self-Love

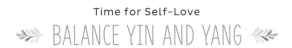

BALANCE YIN AND YANG

In Eastern philosophy, yin and yang are complementary qualities that help us to understand, and achieve, a state of ideal balance. Stray too far in one direction and your lifestyle of beauty, as well as your body, falls out of equilibrium. During the summer season (itself filled with intense yang qualities like heat and bright sunlight), engage in beauty-balancing activities that offer yin qualities like darkness, cool temperatures, dampness, and quiet. Some examples are yin yoga (a restorative, quiet yoga practice), swimming, and walking in the evening when the sun is lower. Modern life is heavily weighted in yang, so choosing yin activities regularly is a route to restoring much-needed balance while addressing your daily need for movement and stress relief.

Beauty Science

PROBIOTICS AND AGING

Add this to the beautifying benefits of probiotic food and supplements: the potential to help your skin age more gracefully. Research has shown that the skin's pH rises as a result of aging; however, one recent study found that probiotics produce acidic molecules that can lower the pH of the skin back to youthful levels. Restoring the skin's naturally acidic pH—and with it, its protective skin barrier—can help it recover more quickly, improve its structure and function, and ward off skin issues like eczema and dermatitis that are associated with higher skin pH. Score one more for the good bacteria.

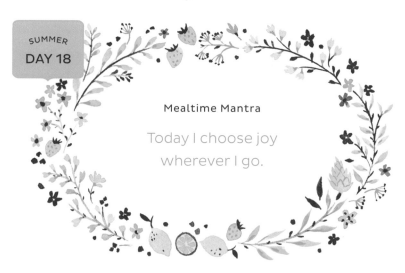

SUMMER
DAY 18

Mealtime Mantra

Today I choose joy
wherever I go.

Kitchen Inspiration

GOODBYE, YELLOWED GREENS

If you've ever bought a beautiful bunch of kale only to find that half of it has yellowed and started to stink before it makes it into your meals, you'll be happy to know that there's a better way. Just look to your freezer. Freezing bunches of greens right after you buy them preserves their nutrition and freshness, which is especially helpful if you are busy and tend to forget to use them while they're at their peak. Wash your greens, from spinach and arugula to kale and green herbs like parsley and basil; pat them dry; and place them in a freezer bag (separate into portions, or discard any thick, tough stems, if you like), then get them right into the freezer. They'll keep weeks longer than they would in the fridge, and, while they won't be useful for salads, you can easily grab them and throw them right into smoothies, soups, and stir-fries.

Intention of the Week

BE PRESENT DURING MEALTIME

Each of us has our own challenges around creating a healthy, beautifying mealtime. Still, there's one particular challenge that I see cropping up again and again: being present and staying focused, rather than distracted with our minds elsewhere, when it's time to eat. What was once a basic right to peaceful focus has become a modern luxury. When we have the opportunity to eat in a relaxed setting, we are more mindful of the way food activates our senses and we are better at eating only what we need to be satisfied. We also allow the body to receive food optimally and recognize signs of fullness earlier. Lunch seems to be the hardest meal to eat mindfully, with the midday spike of phone calls, errands, e-mails, meetings, news, and work assignments. But the body is primed to digest food at this time of day, and a mindful lunch will only enhance that digestive process, giving you a major dose of energy and beauty nutrition that will carry you for hours. This week, try to take a break during mealtimes—especially lunch—and thoroughly enjoy the sight, smells, textures, and flavors of every bite.

Beauty Food Profile

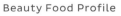 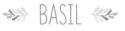

BASIL

Basil, the quintessential summertime herb, is a source of potent antioxidants, including flavonoids that protect your cells and chromosomes from UV radiation and oxidative damage. These fragrant leaves have anti-inflammatory properties that defend against wrinkles and acne; antibacterial oils that boost immunity and fight off foodborne illness; and the phytochemicals lutein and zeaxanthin, which support healthy eyes. Just a small handful of chopped fresh basil contains about a third of your daily recommended vitamin K_1, a nutrient essential for healthy blood vessels. Naturally, freshness counts, so the dried basil in your spice cabinet won't be nearly as beautifying as a big bunch from the farmers' market or just-picked basil from your windowsill garden.

EAT PRETTY FOOD	BEAUTIFYING COMPOUND	BEAUTY BENEFIT
Basil	Flavonoids	Defend against UV radiation

Time for Self-Love
PERK UP WITH A PLANK

Next time you're sitting through a TV commercial, staring at your computer trying to come up with the words to write, or are just plain bored, perk up your body with a "plank" exercise—one of yoga's classic core-strengthening postures. Get down on the floor and hold yourself in the plank pose—push-up position with arms extended, wrists and elbows under your shoulders, back straight, and abs and glutes engaged—for one minute. Next time, try it a little longer; you may find that you break a sweat or your muscles shake from just a few minutes holding this pose! After every round, no matter how long, end by folding back into child's pose with knees bent, shins on the floor, torso lying on top of your thighs, and arms reaching out in front of you, for an extended stretch. Repeat often and you'll have a go-to technique to instantly rev up your focus, increase circulation, and shake off sluggishness. Over time, the plank pose will strengthen your abs and shoulders and support beautiful posture and more relaxed, flexible muscles.

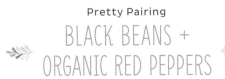

Pretty Pairing

BLACK BEANS +
ORGANIC RED PEPPERS

Why they're more beautiful together: Get more from iron-rich black beans by pairing them with a source of vitamin C like organic red peppers, which increase the body's absorption of plant-based iron. The next time you need an energizing snack, whip up a black bean salsa that includes a generous helping of diced raw red peppers, which retain much higher amounts of vitamin C than roasted peppers.

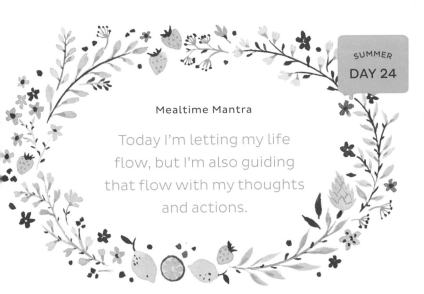

Mealtime Mantra

Today I'm letting my life flow, but I'm also guiding that flow with my thoughts and actions.

Eat Pretty Recipe

❧ SUMMER BEAUTY ELIXIR ❧
ICED RASPBERRY AND ROSE HIP TONIC

*Summer means more time in the sun, so it's absolutely essen-
tial to fill your diet with protective antioxidants and phytochemicals all season long. Of course, you should feel pampered
while you're doing it. Enter this luscious summertime beauty
drink, rich in skin-strengthening anthocyanin pigments and
a megadose of vitamin C from dried rose hips and raw raspberry purée. It's pretty enough to serve in champagne flutes, yet
potent enough to become a new anti-aging staple.*

SERVES 4

4 cups [960 ml] purified water
¼ cup [30 g] whole dried organic
  rose hips (about 30)
1½ cups [170 g] organic
  raspberries

2 Tbsp maple syrup
1 Tbsp water
2 drops liquid stevia

In a saucepan over high heat, bring the water to a boil.
Pack the rose hips into a large heatproof jar and pour
in the hot water. Cover and let steep for 1 to 2 hours, or
until cooled. Strain the infusion and set aside.

    In a high-powered blender, combine the raspberries,
maple syrup, water, and stevia and process until smooth.
Using the back of a spoon, push the purée through a fine-
mesh sieve to remove the seeds. Add the strained purée to
the cooled rose-hip infusion and shake well to combine.
Fill 4 glasses with ice, shake the tonic again, and divide
between the glasses. Serve immediately.

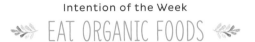

Intention of the Week

EAT ORGANIC FOODS

For the vast majority of us, eating all organic all the time is just plain impossible. You simply can't always ensure that your restaurant salad has a fully organic pedigree, the price of organic groceries often seems prohibitive, and you're not about to refuse your best friend's homemade guacamole because she flavored it with the juice of non-organic limes. But you *can* make a major impact on your exposure to pesticides by opting for organic whenever possible. This week, challenge yourself to buy organic versions of as many of your groceries as you can. After only a short period of organic eating, the pesticide levels in your body could decline sharply. One study showed that after one week of eating at least 80 percent organic foods, urine pesticide levels dropped 89 percent. The presence of pesticides in the body translates to unwanted chemical and free-radical exposures that directly influence your beauty and health. Organic foods also contain higher levels of nutrients—as much as 70 percent higher levels in some foods. For your beauty, the bottom line is less exposure to free radicals, which speed up aging and wrinkling processes, and more beauty nutrition—a complete win-win. At the end of your challenge week, check your grocery bill. You probably spent slightly more, but are those extra few bills a trade-off you're able to make more often? Over time, the beauty and health benefits could add up to far more than what money can buy.

Living Your Best Life
HOW TO INCREASE YOUR HYDRATION

If increasing your water intake is your beauty goal, two easy efforts you can make are eating more water-rich fruits and vegetables like cucumber, apples, melons, tomatoes, and zucchini (since the body hydrates itself while digesting these foods) and drinking more herbal teas, fruit infusions (in which pieces of chopped fruit are added to water), and plain water. To make sipping these liquids a pleasure this summer, choose a pretty pitcher and set it on your desk or on a countertop, wherever you'll see it easily. Keep a glass nearby. Fill the pitcher with your favorite hydrating drink once daily, or more often. Not having to pause and run to the tap makes it easy to throw back an extra glass or two while you go about your day.

Kitchen Inspiration

ENERGY-BOOSTING FOODS

You've been there before—you're feeling particularly low in energy, like you could use an extra dose of *something* to help you get through the day. What do you reach for? (Hint: it's not a shot of espresso.) Create space in your kitchen for three important categories of energy-boosting beauty foods: 1) Super-concentrated sources of nutrition like bee pollen, spirulina, and chia or hemp seeds (perfect for tossing into a smoothie); 2) foods that will keep your blood sugar stable and give you long-lasting energy, like avocados, raw nuts, lentils, and coconut oil (think, a lentil salad, raw trail mix, or avocado with a dash of salt and spices); and 3) energy-enhancing superfoods like cacao, maca, or green tea to rev you up with phytochemical power (sip a cup of green tea or whip up a maca hot cocoa). These foods are all strongly energizing and beautifying to your body, and free of the negative effects of an afternoon caffeine jolt.

Beauty Science
STRESS AND DIGESTION

You already know stress can give you a tension headache, or sap your energy. But, says one recent study, it can also interfere with the way you break down and absorb your beauty nutrition. Stress destroys the good bacteria in our guts, while simultaneously helping the bad bacteria to take hold. Those lost good bacteria are critical for immunity, healthy weight, and radiant skin, as well as aging well overall. So the next time you take a break to breathe, laugh, or exercise away stress, remember that you're doing it for a flat belly and glowing skin as much as to relieve that fleeting headache.

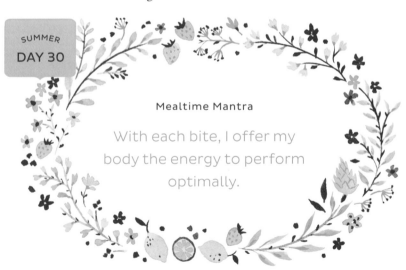

Mealtime Mantra

With each bite, I offer my body the energy to perform optimally.

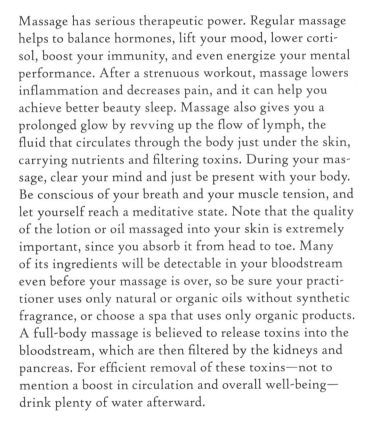

Time for Self-Love

BREAK FOR MASSAGE THERAPY

Massage has serious therapeutic power. Regular massage helps to balance hormones, lift your mood, lower cortisol, boost your immunity, and even energize your mental performance. After a strenuous workout, massage lowers inflammation and decreases pain, and it can help you achieve better beauty sleep. Massage also gives you a prolonged glow by revving up the flow of lymph, the fluid that circulates through the body just under the skin, carrying nutrients and filtering toxins. During your massage, clear your mind and just be present with your body. Be conscious of your breath and your muscle tension, and let yourself reach a meditative state. Note that the quality of the lotion or oil massaged into your skin is extremely important, since you absorb it from head to toe. Many of its ingredients will be detectable in your bloodstream even before your massage is over, so be sure your practitioner uses only natural or organic oils without synthetic fragrance, or choose a spa that uses only organic products. A full-body massage is believed to release toxins into the bloodstream, which are then filtered by the kidneys and pancreas. For efficient removal of these toxins—not to mention a boost in circulation and overall well-being— drink plenty of water afterward.

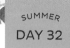
Beauty Food Profile

SUNFLOWER SEEDS

Sunflower seeds are bursting with good-for-you fats and beauty minerals that nourish radiant, dewy skin. They're high in iron, zinc, copper, and phosphorus, a range of minerals that support immunity, nervous function, and energy. They're also excellent sources of plant-based protein and free radical–fighting, skin- and scalp-hydrating vitamin E. Additionally, sunflower seeds contain significant amounts of calming magnesium and an impressive range of B vitamins that maintain healthy hair and supple skin, and aid in cell growth and repair. Buy yours raw and unsalted, and store them in the refrigerator to keep their fats in top form.

EAT PRETTY FOOD	BEAUTIFYING COMPOUND	BEAUTY BENEFIT
Sunflower seeds	Healthy fat	Strengthens cell membranes and skin barrier

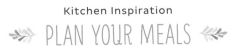

Kitchen Inspiration

PLAN YOUR MEALS

As much fun as it is to go to the farmers' market and fill your basket with the foods that happen to inspire you in the moment, meals don't always fall together effortlessly when you've brought home a bunch of random ingredients (especially if you're just learning how to cook without a recipe). It helps to have at least a few seasonal meals in mind *before* you hit the market or grocery store, so you make it home with the ingredients you need for two or three meals. Once you've gathered those ingredients, then fill in with others that you get excited about. To keep ideas at the ready, post a list of your favorite meals, sides, and snacks on the side of your fridge. You can organize them seasonally, or adjust them slightly to fit ingredients that are available and in season. That way, you'll never be completely lost for beautifying meal ideas, and you'll have a place to keep track of meals that you want to repeat again and again.

Intention of the Week

BRING NEW COLORS INTO YOUR DIET AND YOUR EATING SPACE

Even after we've established healthy, feel-good habits, we can still easily get bored with a routine that never changes, from gym to journal to cooking. This week, for your Eat Pretty practice, take time to wake up your senses by infusing mealtime with new doses of color. Shop for, cook, and eat a true rainbow of fruits and vegetables—you might even have fun focusing on one color each day this week to make sure you get to them all—to assure a wide range of nutrients, phytochemicals, and antioxidants in your diet. To go further, bring colorful flowers to your table to create a space where peace and presence prevails. Then let yourself slow down, taste, and see the colorful feast for eyes, mind, and body you've created at mealtime.

Time for Self-Love

SEEK A CHANGE OF SCENERY

Travel, whether to a neighboring city or across the globe, provides a change of perspective that helps you reflect on your daily routine. What makes that so valuable for your beauty? Not only can that opportunity for reflection inspire big changes, renewed focus on your priorities, and priceless inspiration to live life to its fullest, it can also allow for a new perspective when you look in the mirror. Seeing yourself in a new place lets you look beyond perceived flaws and see the adventurous, beautiful person you are, inside and out!

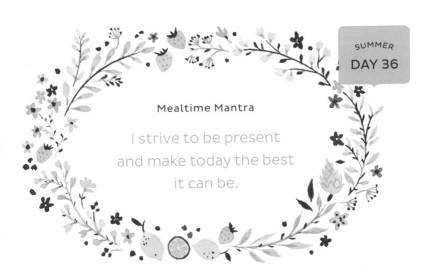

Mealtime Mantra

I strive to be present and make today the best it can be.

Living Your Best Life

HOW TO GLOW WITH GRATITUDE

Gratitude: it's the key to a glass-half-full view of life. When you flex your positivity muscle by consciously expressing gratitude for life's moments, big and small, you increase your happiness and the good-mood neurotransmitters serotonin and dopamine; you develop resilience; you grow in attractiveness to others; and—I strongly believe—you deepen your overall glow, from radiant skin to sparkling eyes. Beauty from gratitude and positivity is not something that's quantifiable in a lab test, but it only takes a minute, for example, to consider the people you find most beautiful and to appreciate that their positivity contributes to their magnetism. Today, make a short list of things you're grateful for, from a lovingly prepared meal, to a few extra minutes to sit outside and enjoy the twilight, to the cool breeze blowing the moisture from your face. Feel grateful for the beauty all around and within you.

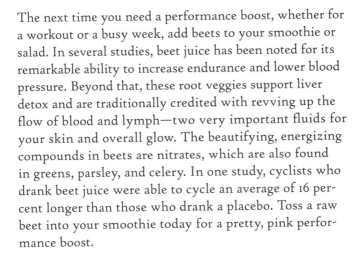

Kitchen Inspiration

PERFORM BETTER WITH BEETS

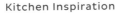

The next time you need a performance boost, whether for a workout or a busy week, add beets to your smoothie or salad. In several studies, beet juice has been noted for its remarkable ability to increase endurance and lower blood pressure. Beyond that, these root veggies support liver detox and are traditionally credited with revving up the flow of blood and lymph—two very important fluids for your skin and overall glow. The beautifying, energizing compounds in beets are nitrates, which are also found in greens, parsley, and celery. In one study, cyclists who drank beet juice were able to cycle an average of 16 percent longer than those who drank a placebo. Toss a raw beet into your smoothie today for a pretty, pink performance boost.

Eat Pretty Recipe

SWEET SUMMER TREAT

CHERRY-ALMOND CHIA JAM

This naturally sweet jam will satisfy your biggest sweet crav-ings while serving as a beautifying alternative to jams and jellies made with loads of refined sugar. A spoonful pairs well with nut butter, and it's a perfect add-in for oatmeal. Anthocy-anins in the skins of cherries protect your skin's elasticity, while chia seeds offer nourishing omega fats and cinnamon helps to offset the age-advancing spike in blood sugar that you get from all sugars.

MAKES ABOUT 1 CUP [10 OZ/280 G]

2 cups [280 g] halved, pitted
  organic sweet cherries
1 Tbsp maple syrup
2 Tbsp chia seeds

½ tsp ground cinnamon
A few drops of organic almond
  extract

In a saucepan, heat the cherries and maple syrup until the mixture begins to bubble, stirring occasionally. Reduce the heat to maintain a low simmer. Using a spoon, break apart the cherries and press them against the side of the pot to release their juices.

Stir in the chia seeds and cinnamon and simmer until the jam thickens, about 10 minutes, continuing to mash the cherries and stir frequently. When the jam has thickened, remove from the heat and let cool. Stir in the almond extract. Store in an airtight container in the refrigerator for up to 1 week.

Intention of the Week

EXPLORE BEAUTY-FRIENDLY ALTERNATIVES TO BREAD

Bread has earned a bad rap for being nutritionally bland and often full of Beauty Betrayers (see page 10). I find that bread is one food that my clients are especially worried and confused about cutting back on, but with just a little effort, you can find a handful of beauty nutrition–packed bread alternatives that are easy to include in your meal rotation. You'll likely be excited when you discover fresh, new ways to eat a sandwich! Experiment with a few this week. For starters, try wrapping your sandwiches in large lettuce, cabbage, or collard green leaves, perfect for celebrating summer. Try rolling up ingredients in nori seaweed sheets or brown rice–paper wrappers. Even grilled slices of eggplant or tempeh can keep your sandwich in place. Sure, they're not exactly close cousins of crusty sandwich bread, but they pack in way more beauty nutrition, add interest to your plate, and can earn you some extra culinary cred.

Pretty Pairing
❧ PINEAPPLE + ALMOND BUTTER ❧

Why they're more beautiful together: For a fresh and beauty-friendly pairing, slather sweet chunks of pineapple with creamy almond butter, or blend the two into a sweet smoothie with a splash of coconut milk. Almond butter contains healthy fats and protein that slow the absorption of pineapple's natural sugar to reduce the resulting blood sugar spike, while pineapple's powerful anti-inflammatory enzyme bromelain helps break down the protein in almond butter so you digest it more fully.

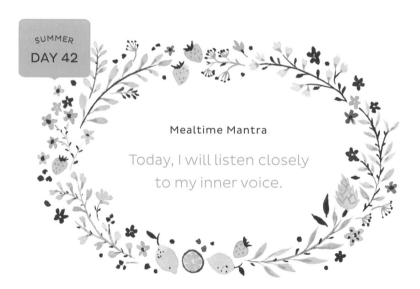

Mealtime Mantra

Today, I will listen closely
to my inner voice.

Beauty Food Profile

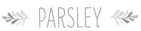 PARSLEY

Parsley is an anti-inflammatory, detoxifying herb that freshens breath (thanks to its chlorophyll and anti-bacterial properties), reduces water retention, supports liver and kidney health, and aids in blood sugar and hormone balance. Parsley, like many other green herbs, promotes healthy digestion by warding off bad bacteria in the gut. It stimulates production of anti-aging gluta-thione in the body, protecting the mitochondria and oxygenating the blood. Nutritionally, parsley is a great source of iron (over 10 percent of your daily need in a big handful) and is incredibly high in vitamin K_1 (almost 600 percent in the same amount), which strengthens healthy blood vessels. I regularly add a handful, stems and all, to my green smoothies for fresh, bright flavor and mega nutrition.

EAT PRETTY FOOD	BEAUTIFYING COMPOUND	BEAUTY BENEFIT
Parsley	Iron	Supports hair, nails, and energy

Kitchen Inspiration

EAT PREBIOTICS

"Prebiotics," probably less well-known than probiotics but rapidly gaining name recognition, are fiber compounds that feed probiotic bacteria, keeping them happy and thriving in your digestive tract. While prebiotics are, like probiotics, available in capsules that can be ingested and powders that can be added to food, you can also get them directly from your diet. Meals packed with beauty foods happen to be an excellent foundation for the prebiotics that complement a healthy gut (and clear, glowing skin). Specific prebiotic-rich beauty foods include asparagus, bananas, chicories, garlic, greens, oats, onions, leeks, and sunchokes.

Time for Self-Love

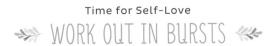 WORK OUT IN BURSTS

Endurance is prized in the world of exercise, and so many of us log countless hours at the gym trying to lose weight and achieve our perfect body by tacking on longer and longer challenges. And of course it's common for celebrities to credit three- or four-hour daily workouts for their ability to stay red-carpet ready. While setting big fitness goals is a beauty *do*, the frequency with which you exercise may actually be more important than the total hours you log burning calories. There's evidence that dedicating your entire evening to the gym may not produce the results you want it to—plus it could wind up contributing to hormonal issues in the form of adrenal burnout, especially if you already have a lot of stress in your life. While you may be eager to take on the challenge of a long workout at times, give yourself permission to log a shorter workout—a ten-minute jog here, a five-minute weight session there, maybe a few push-ups to get your circulation pumping—more often, especially if long workouts sap your motivation. The takeaway here is that only you can decide what workout your body needs—but don't believe that it's not worth lacing up your sneakers at all if you can't commit to a long session.

Intention of the Week

FOCUS ON YOUR FAVORITE THING IN THE MIRROR

When you look at a friend or loved one, do you seek out their flaws, or are you drawn to the qualities that make them beautiful, like sparkling eyes or a warm smile? We seem to find it easy to admire the beautiful characteristics of others, but are quick to home in on our own flaws when we look in a mirror. This week, instead of focusing on the blemish on your cheek or the circles under your eyes when you look in the mirror, take note of the trait you love most. Look at your reflection and draw your eyes right to your silky, glossy hair or your cute, one-of-a-kind nose. Appreciate them and use them to rev up your confidence, and, when you step out from behind the mirror, trust that others see your positive traits as well.

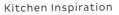

Kitchen Inspiration
REVERSE TRADITIONAL PORTIONS

When planning your next meal or filling your plate, consider reversing traditional mealtime roles, in which meat is the focus and vegetables are the side dishes. Let vegetables take center stage, and fill in the gaps with smaller portions of fish, eggs, and plant-based proteins like quinoa or tempeh (or other organic animal meats if you choose to eat them). Aim to fill more than half of your plate with vegetable-based dishes, then take note of the way your body feels after making this antioxidant-boosting switch.

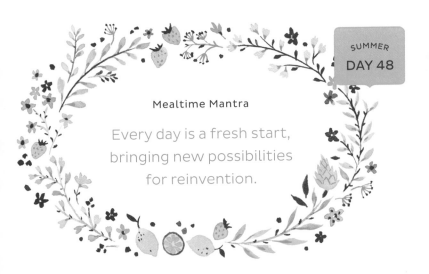

Mealtime Mantra

Every day is a fresh start,
bringing new possibilities
for reinvention.

Eat Pretty Recipe

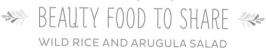

BEAUTY FOOD TO SHARE

WILD RICE AND ARUGULA SALAD

This is a perfect picnic or potluck salad—one that provides a beautifying, delicious, and allergen-free option for a crowd. Wild rice, not a grain but actually a grass, is a true beauty food high in protein, fiber, and minerals like iron, and also offers anti-inflammatory omega-3s.

SERVES 4 TO 6

3 cups [490 g] cooked wild rice

1 heaping cup [150 g] halved and pitted olives (I like Castelvetrano)

1 heaping cup [200 g] halved organic cherry or grape tomatoes

3 scallions, white and crisp green parts only, finely chopped

¼ cup [60 ml] olive oil

2 Tbsp apple cider vinegar

1 tsp dried oregano

Unrefined salt and freshly ground black pepper

2 large handfuls baby arugula

In a large serving bowl, combine the wild rice, olives, tomatoes, and scallions and toss to mix. In a small bowl, whisk together the olive oil, vinegar, oregano, and salt and pepper to taste. Pour the dressing over the salad and toss gently to coat. Just before serving, toss in the arugula.

Beauty Science
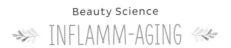
INFLAMM-AGING

Inflammation is a natural bodily response that can be helpful to your body in the moment—but harmful when it lasts and lasts. "Inflamm-aging" is a term for the link between prolonged, low-level inflammation and age-associated concerns like wrinkles, redness, weight gain, dryness, and textural changes in our skin. Cosmetic research has identified inflammation to be one of the biggest factors in aging, hence the ability of anti-inflammatory foods like ginger, turmeric, pomegranate, olive oil, and green tea (to name just a few) to help you age more slowly and beautifully. Topically, studies show that anti-inflammatory foods and botanicals like oats and green tea also calm surface inflammation. Now you know why focusing on "anti-inflammatory" means more beauty in the mirror.

Living Your Best Life

HOW TO BUY THE SAFEST SEAFOOD

When buying fish, it's essential to look into the source to make sure you're getting the most beautifying varieties. Concern continues to grow about toxins found in fish and other seafood (the beauty benefits get canceled out if you're also getting exposed to mercury or other toxic compounds), as well as about depleted populations; however, if you do your homework and make conscious choices, you'll find plenty of clean and sustainable fish to add to your beauty diet. Here are three things to keep in mind when you shop: 1) You will often find that the cleanest, most nutritious fish costs more, like wild salmon instead of farmed salmon. If you are concerned that you can't afford the higher-quality kind, consider purchasing a smaller portion that fits your budget rather than compromising on quality. 2) Seek sources lower on the food chain, like sardines, oysters, and anchovies, for less toxins and greater sustainability. 3) Look for guides and apps that stay up to the moment with changing info. The news on fish continues to develop, so find a continuously updated source that you can refer to easily when you shop.

Time for Self-Love

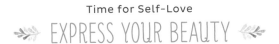 EXPRESS YOUR BEAUTY

You know, of course, that your clothes and the items in your makeup bag don't define your beauty. But many of us enjoy using them as tools for expressing—and accentuating—the unique qualities that make us gorgeous. If done in a loving way, the time we spend dressing ourselves and applying makeup can be a valuable investment in our beauty. Assess the tools you are currently using to express yourself through your appearance. Do the colors in your makeup bag and the clothes in your closet align with the best self you want to show to the world? Do they reflect your unique style—one that you might describe as effortless, striking, avant-garde, au naturel, etc.? What might need to change to ensure that you are expressing your most beautiful, authentic self every day? Practice letting the way you present yourself to the world complement and play off of the unique qualities that you love most about yourself.

Beauty Science

A SUN-PROTECTIVE DIET

Want to give your skin extra sun-defense abilities this summer? Increase the lycopene, beta-carotene, and omega-3s in your diet. Studies have shown that all three of these nutrients decrease our susceptibility to sunburn after UV exposure. Try a meal of wild salmon (a great source of omega-3s), steamed spinach (which contains beta-carotene), and tomatoes (excellent sources of lycopene), drizzled in olive oil to increase your nutrient absorption, for a triple sun protection boost from the inside out.

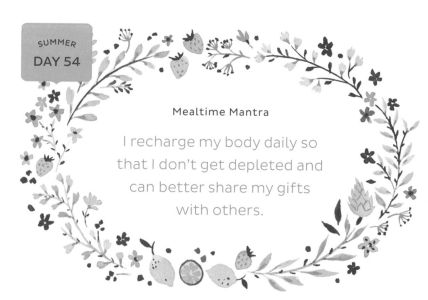

Mealtime Mantra

I recharge my body daily so that I don't get depleted and can better share my gifts with others.

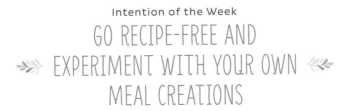

Intention of the Week
GO RECIPE-FREE AND EXPERIMENT WITH YOUR OWN MEAL CREATIONS

One of my favorite cooking shows challenges chefs to create a meal that incorporates a basketful of mismatched, odd ingredients. When I'm low on groceries and I open my cabinets or fridge, I'm playing that game in my head: what beauty nutrition–packed meal can I make from the random ingredients, leftovers, and other bits and pieces I have to work with today? This week, I challenge you to play, too. Create a few new recipes that come from your head and your palate, rather than a cookbook. (Keep in mind that this measurement-free method works best for simple entrées and sides like soups, stews, sautés, and salads—but not always baked goods!) There is no faster way to get comfortable cooking with beauty foods than to take charge of their flavors on your own. I'm betting you encounter a few winning combinations that make it into your regular repertoire.

Kitchen Inspiration

HOMEMADE ALOE VERA DRINKS

Aloe vera is a medicinal plant with powerful internal and external healing properties. It's been said to soothe the digestive tract, reduce inflammation, regulate elimination, and, of course, heal wounds. You may have seen trendy aloe waters and aloe beauty drinks sold in stores, but you can easily make your own versions at home. Cut away the green outer skin from either a small piece of organic aloe purchased from a farmers' market or a small, pesticide-free piece of aloe leaf grown in your home, keeping the jellylike insides. Alternatively, purchase a concentrated bottle of pure, organic aloe juice from a store. Add just a small amount (1 to 2 Tbsp) of the gel or juice to smoothies at the very end of your smoothie recipe, taking care to blend it minimally. (Store any excess aloe in the fridge for later.) A couple of things to keep in mind before incorporating aloe into your diet: Aloe has a strong taste to go along with its strong benefits, and many find it easier to consume when there are other flavors present. Also, since ingesting aloe can cause upset stomachs for some people, talk to your doctor before you give it a try.

Time for Self-Love

REDEFINE A BEAUTIFYING WORKOUT

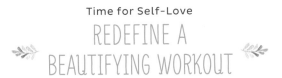

Great workouts don't feel like exercise. And some of the *best* workouts are the ones that challenge your body while helping you give back. You will do your mind and body an even greater favor by seeking ways to occasionally swap your regular workout for a project that needs volunteers and involves physical activity, like a beach cleanup, park construction, or house-building for those in need. If you can't find a group to join, look around you to find a place that needs beautifying; get your hands dirty while you break a sweat planting flowers or cutting grass. You'll test your body in new ways and work out your emotional wellness while building beauty in your body and in the world around you.

Beauty Food Profile
TART CHERRIES

The sweet cherries that hit the farmers' market in the summer are tasty, beautiful, and easy to love. But there's a different variety of cherry—the tart cherry, or sour cherry—that holds even more potent beauty benefits in its slightly tangier taste. Tart cherries rank as one of the top foods for both antioxidant levels and anti-inflammatory compounds—two incredible boosters for beauty and radiant skin. At least one study suggests that their anti-inflammatory benefits rival those of over-the-counter anti-inflammatory drugs. Tart cherries rank far higher than sweet cherries in anthocyanins, which boost skin elasticity, and they contain both melatonin and tryptophan, which help with beauty sleep. These beautifying cherries, which also contain both skin-healing vitamin A and energy-supporting iron, are available fresh in the summer and dried year-round. Add a few to your morning smoothie or cereal, or grab a small handful of dried, unsweetened cherries and raw nuts for a sweet snack.

EAT PRETTY FOOD	BEAUTIFYING COMPOUND	BEAUTY BENEFIT
Tart cherries	Anthocyanins	Boost skin elasticity

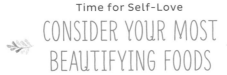

Time for Self-Love

CONSIDER YOUR MOST BEAUTIFYING FOODS

As you've learned more about beauty nutrition, you've been listening to your body and taking note of how it responds to certain foods. Pop quiz: Which food or foods have delivered the most beautifying benefits to you lately? What beauty food is your body craving right now? Quite often we find that one or two particular foods really resonate with our body and fulfill needs that we might not have even been aware of. Notice when a beauty food really hits the spot—and give it a regular place on your grocery list so you can get your fill.

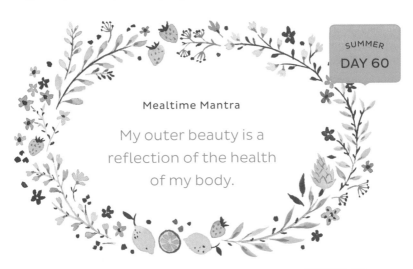

Mealtime Mantra

My outer beauty is a reflection of the health of my body.

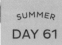

Beauty Science

MEALS WITH FRIENDS

Studies show that when dining with friends, we tend to make poor food choices if our friends make them as well. But there's another side to this observation: if we, or our friends, make healthy choices, then the whole group is apt to eat healthier! Start sharing your beauty nutrition–packed meals with friends who have the same goal of looking and feeling their best. The result could be that you eat healthier more often, along with your besties. To deepen the benefits, spend time in the kitchen together. Share ingredients. Swap culinary tips. Then sit down to a meal where you are relaxed and present. The food is nourishing, the social connection builds happiness, and the beauty benefits will keep you coming back again and again.

Intention of the Week

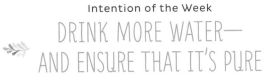

DRINK MORE WATER— AND ENSURE THAT IT'S PURE

Most of us don't drink enough water daily, which means that the simple act of consuming more of it can have profound beauty benefits. Adequate hydration is essential for nutrient absorption, metabolism, detoxification, circulation, and temperature regulation—and water makes up about 70 percent of our skin. While you're increasing your H_2O intake this week, challenge yourself to get to know what's in the water that you drink, whether it comes from your well or tap, local springs, or purchased bottles. It's easy and affordable to buy a drinking-water test kit to detect exactly what's in your primary water source, and there are many water authorities that can provide this info for you if you do a little digging into local resources. If need be, invest in a filter to ensure that you're not regularly ingesting unnecessary toxins, from byproducts of chlorination, hormones, and antibiotics to minerals from pipes and the soil. A glass of water is a precious resource, and even more valuable in its purest form.

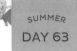
Living Your Best Life

HOW TO KICK A SODA ADDICTION

Some of my clients come to me willing to do anything to improve their skin, energy, and overall beauty—except give up soda. Together, we work on getting these ultra-sweet, age-advancing beverages (the high levels of phosphates in soda have been linked to skin aging and tooth and bone decay, and soda consumption is also tied to a wrinkle-promoting process in the body) out of their regular routines by including more herbal teas, lemon water, and fizzy, fermented drinks like kombucha and water kefir. All four of these beverages offer beauty benefits, but I find that the fermented drinks often have the most success in replacing soda once and for all. Fermented kombuchas and water kefirs have varying contents of sugar and liquid calories (meaning they're *still* a treat), so look carefully at labels and choose wisely, but do try one next time you're about to reach for a can of cola. You may find that a bubbly, refreshing fermented drink kicks your craving for soda, while delivering a healthful dose of probiotic bacteria.

Eat Pretty Recipe

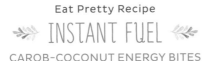# INSTANT FUEL

CAROB-COCONUT ENERGY BITES

These sweet, chewy bites combine the skin-beautifying fats and instantly usable fuel of coconut with protein-packed almonds. Carob powder, ground from the pods and delivering rich, toasty flavor, also adds calcium and fiber to these super-portable and satisfying snacks. One or two will rev up your energy and satisfy a sweet tooth without refined sugar.

MAKES ABOUT 12 BITES

⅓ cup [55 g] pitted dates, soaked in hot water to cover for 10 minutes

1 cup [100 g] almond meal (finely ground almonds)

2 Tbsp coconut oil

2 Tbsp toasted carob powder

2 Tbsp unsweetened coconut flakes

⅛ tsp unrefined salt

Drain and finely chop the soaked dates. Combine all of the ingredients in a food processor and pulse until the mixture is well blended. Roll into 1-in [2.5-cm] balls. Store in an airtight container in the refrigerator for up to one week.

Kitchen Inspiration

SUMMER SMOOTHIE ENHANCERS

During the summer, you're frequently in motion, whether traveling, spending time outdoors, or socializing with friends and family. To look and feel your best this season, you need energy and antioxidants that will protect and enhance your beauty. Add these beautifying foods to a smoothie for energizing fuel and beauty on the go this summer: coconut oil and chia, for energy and fullness; fresh herbs like basil, mint, and parsley, for antioxidant benefits; and maca, for hormone balance. Incorporate one or more of these ingredients in your favorite smoothie recipes for an extra dose of summer beauty nutrition.

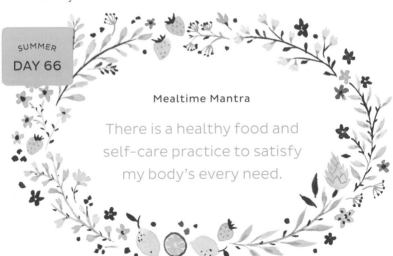

Mealtime Mantra

There is a healthy food and self-care practice to satisfy my body's every need.

Intention of the Week

EXPLORE BEAUTIFYING ALTERNATIVES TO YOUR AVERAGE GRAINS

Sometimes making our diets more beautifying is as easy as instituting creative ingredient swaps in recipes we already know and love. This week, I challenge you to look past the grains you reach for again and again, like much-used wheat, corn, oats, and rice, and try a grain with even greater beauty benefits. Even if you don't replace your old standbys completely, you'll be livening up your palate and varying your nutritional benefits. If you usually stir-fry veggies and toss them with pasta, mix them into quinoa instead. If you serve rice as a side dish, replace it with buckwheat. And if corn polenta is your staple, try teff polenta in its place. Other grains to experiment with include millet, amaranth, wild rice, and black rice. Interestingly, quinoa, millet, buckwheat, wild rice, and amaranth are actually seeds, although we eat them like grains, just one reason that they help bring nutritional diversity to our diets.

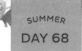
Beauty Food Profile

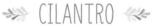

CILANTRO

While its flavor can be polarizing, cilantro deserves a regular place on our plates and in our beauty smoothies for its powerful detox and digestive benefits. Cilantro is traditionally revered for its ability to detoxify the body, especially from heavy metals, making it a go-to ingredient in many juice cleanses. But cilantro's benefits extend to the digestive system, where it reduces inflammation, nausea, gas, bloating, water retention, and digestive pain, and supports healthy digestion overall, perhaps in part due to its natural antibacterial qualities. Though cilantro is usually eaten in small amounts, it still packs a major antioxidant punch from an array of anti-aging phytochemicals like quercetin and kaempferol, as well as a nice dose of vitamin A.

EAT PRETTY FOOD	BEAUTIFYING COMPOUND	BEAUTY BENEFIT
Cilantro	Kaempferol	Blocks wrinkle formation

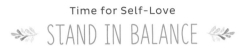

Time for Self-Love

STAND IN BALANCE

One of the most important physical skills to cultivate in order to age gracefully is our ability to balance. At any age, it's never too early or late to get in the habit of strengthening and challenging your balance skills so they don't weaken. If you're a yoga devotee, poses like one-legged tree or half moon work on your balance muscles, but you can also tune up your balance with simple exercises you integrate into your daily routine. Give yourself balance challenges as you go about your day (those boring moments while we are brushing our teeth or folding laundry are great opportunities) by standing on one leg and extending the other leg in front or behind you. Bend the knee of your standing leg for an extra challenge. Surprisingly, simply walking barefoot can also support lifelong balance by awakening receptors in your feet that send signals to your brain. The bonus from all of this one-legged time is better muscle tone today and fewer falls in the future.

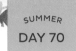

Kitchen Inspiration

PLAY WITH PESTO

Beyond its intense burst of flavor, traditional pesto has amazing beauty benefits, from the concentrated anti-inflammatory phytochemicals in the basil to wrinkle-blocking allicin in the garlic to skin-nourishing healthy fats in the olive oil and pine nuts. But pesto doesn't have to be built the same way every time, and alternative versions can really break the mold and freshen up your cooking. To make a variation on pesto, keep the classic pesto formula intact (no cheese needed), but substitute similar ingredients for the olive oil, basil, and pine nuts. Use a flavored oil like sesame or avocado in place of olive. Replace basil with spicy watercress or arugula, beautifying kale and parsley, garlicky ramps, or a blend of your favorite greens. Swap in walnuts, almonds, cashews, or even pumpkin seeds for the pine nuts. Add unrefined salt and black pepper and pulse in a food processor until smooth. You'll have concentrated beauty nutrition in each rich, savory bite.

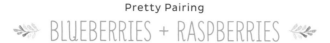

Pretty Pairing

BLUEBERRIES + RASPBERRIES

Why they're more beautiful together: Berries are among the highest sources of antioxidant phytochemicals. Combine blueberries and raspberries and you'll not only have a snack that's beautiful on the eyes, but you'll also enhance the power of their individual anti-aging compounds, since the phytochemicals in these berries strengthen each other's beautifying properties.

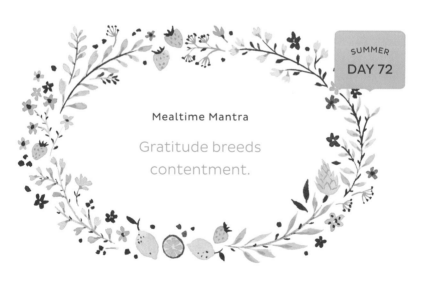

Mealtime Mantra

Gratitude breeds
contentment.

Intention of the Week

❧ PICK YOUR OWN BEAUTY FOODS ☙

Pulling tomatoes right off the vine or berries from the patch is an amazing—yet increasingly rare—experience. But summer offers a special chance to do so, if you seek out local farms that let you get right in their fields and gardens to harvest your own peaches, peppers, eggplant, blueberries, and many of the other beautifying foods available this season. Eating just-picked produce is the ultimate luxury! This week, find an opportunity to let your hands do the picking and your skin do the celebrating. While you're at it, pick *more* than you need and store some away for the colder months. You can freeze trays of juicy peach slices or blueberries (transfer to freezer bags or containers after the fruits are individually frozen) to be enjoyed over fall oatmeal, or preserve tomatoes (you can hot-pack can them in a water bath, or roast them, cool them, and then freeze them in glass containers) that will spice up a winter chili. Freezing and canning are two ways to extend nature's beauty benefits, even out of season.

Beauty Food Profile

MULBERRIES

Mulberries may seem like a hot new superfruit, but they've been around for centuries. The bark of the mulberry tree was used to make currency in China during the time of Marco Polo. Today we know that mulberries are one of the rare fruits packed with protein and iron, plus a range of B-complex vitamins essential for keeping your hair, nails, and skin healthy and strong. Like red grapes, mulberries contain the antioxidant phytochemical resveratrol, which may help with blood sugar control and free-radical defense. The potent dose of vitamin C (plus protein) in mulberries is key for building collagen, while its flavonoids keep your immune system strong. As a bonus, look out for mulberry leaf tea, a caffeine-free herbal brew that offers an antioxidant boost and supports steady blood sugar and healthy liver function.

EAT PRETTY FOOD	BEAUTIFYING COMPOUND	BEAUTY BENEFIT
Mulberries	Resveratrol	Defends against free radicals

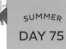

Kitchen Inspiration

HEALTHY DESSERT TOPPINGS

Who doesn't love sprinkles? Sadly, their rainbow hues offer beauty, but no benefits. Next time you feel like adding a decorative topping, or some extra texture, to your favorite pudding, smoothie, or coconut ice cream, reach for hemp seeds, raw cocoa nibs, or bee pollen. All three toothsome add-ins supercharge the beauty nutrition in your dessert. Hemp seeds are one of my top picks for protein (an absolute must for healthy hair), while raw cocoa nibs provide major antioxidants and mood-boosting alkaloids, and bee pollen (skip this one if you have bee allergies) is packed with enzymes that energize your body.

Living Your Best Life

HOW TO REDUCE PESTICIDES IN YOUR HOME ENVIRONMENT

Pesticides can increase the free-radical burden in your body, speeding up the aging process as well as making it harder for you to maintain a healthy weight. But even if you buy all organic foods, you still could be surrounded by pesticides at home. One easy way to reduce unwanted germs, allergens, pesticides, and other toxins that end up being tracked into your home environment from lawns, parks, streets, and public floors is to remove your shoes while indoors. This simple act can dramatically reduce the amount of toxins that end up floating around your home, being breathed in or coming into contact with your skin. Make your home a sacred space by removing your shoes right away, and you'll be supporting a healthy beauty and body.

Time for Self-Love

FEEL ALIVE—AND AMAZING

Today, take a moment to appreciate, and feel, that you are alive. What allows us to feel so vital in the summer? We sweat from every pore, feel the sun's rays sear our skin, slip bare feet into plush grass, and soak up every last drop of sunlight from the day. No matter what your age, situation, or struggle at the moment, you're here—and it's a gift. Summer is the season not only to appreciate that you are alive and beautiful, but to put a little life back into your days. Cultivate a youthful, refreshed mindset and you'll glow just a little more as well.

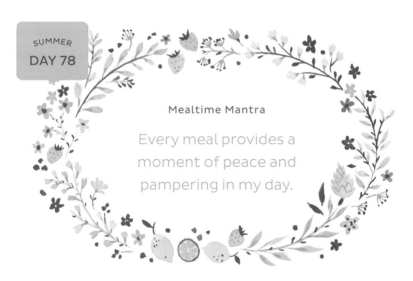

Mealtime Mantra

Every meal provides a moment of peace and pampering in my day.

Eat Pretty Recipe

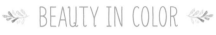

BEAUTY IN COLOR

RAINBOW SUMMER SALAD WITH
LEMON-OREGANO DRESSING

*The beautiful colors of this rainbow-hued salad will draw you
in, while its concentrated beauty benefits and the freshness
of its oregano-scented dressing will lure you back for seconds.
Feel free to add in any fresh vegetables you have on hand to
suit your beauty nutrition needs of the moment.*

SERVES 4

5 oz [140 g] chopped mixed greens (try romaine, arugula, and chard)

1 organic tomato, cut into wedges

1 small yellow squash, trimmed and sliced lengthwise into very thin ribbons

1 organic orange bell pepper, seeded and chopped

⅓ cup [80 ml] extra-virgin olive oil

2 Tbsp fresh organic lemon juice, plus zest of ½ organic lemon

1 heaping Tbsp fresh oregano leaves, minced

1 clove garlic, minced

Unrefined salt and freshly ground black pepper

¼ cup [30 g] shelled hemp seeds

In a large serving bowl, combine the greens, tomato,
squash, and bell pepper and toss to mix. In a high-powered
blender or mini food processor, combine the olive oil,
lemon juice and zest, oregano, garlic, and salt and pepper
to taste, and process until the garlic and oregano are finely
chopped, about 1 minute. Pour the dressing over the salad
(you may not need all of it) and toss gently to coat. Sprinkle with the hemp seeds and serve immediately.

Kitchen Inspiration
ALL-IN-ONE SNACKS

A piece of fruit makes a great snack because it's portable and requires no prep to enjoy. But couldn't you say the same about vegetables? Look beyond apples and bananas and discover other convenient snack options in colorful, nutrient-dense vegetables. This summer, stock up on organic cucumbers, bell peppers, carrots, celery, and green beans, all ready to wash, trim, and grab—and go, if needed. Add hummus or nut butter for bonus protein. Sure, it's a bit unexpected to pull a pepper out of your purse, but like an apple, it's crisp, satisfying, and surprisingly easy to enjoy on the go. And really, who can argue with a gorgeous fresh veggie—and the radiant skin that goes with it?

Beauty Food Profile

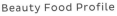 OREGANO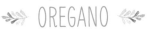

This flavorful plant appears to have the highest anti-oxidant capacity of any herb, plus a strong ability to eliminate bacteria, viruses, fungus, and parasites from the body. It's prized for its ability to aid in the prevention and healing of infection and illness, especially issues that arise in the gut. Oregano is even more powerful than garlic at destroying bacteria like salmonella, e. coli, and listeria that cause food poisoning, which may be due to its anti-bacterial phytochemicals thymol and carvacrol. In addition to using fresh and dried oregano in your meals, oregano oil is often used, diluted and in very small doses, as an immune and digestive strengthener that wards off candida yeast in the body.

EAT PRETTY FOOD	BEAUTIFYING COMPOUND	BEAUTY BENEFIT
Oregano	Thymol	Destroys unwanted bacteria

Intention of the Week

FILL YOUR DIET WITH ALKALINE FOODS

There's a beautifying, alternative way to balance your diet that starts with the pH scale. The internal environment of our bodies operates at a slightly alkaline pH, which is influenced by our diet and daily habits. Problem is, the vast majority of the foods we eat create acid inside our bodies! This week, eat more alkaline foods, like green vegetables, lemons and limes (which are acidic to our tongues but have an alkaline effect in the body), and most fruits, herbs, and spices, to balance out acidic beauty foods like grains and nuts. While you're at it, make an effort to cut back on acidic foods that aren't helping your skin, from dairy and caffeine to meats and sugar. You can also balance your pH with the seasons, by loading up on alkaline veggies when they're fresh in the spring, summer, and early fall. When late fall and winter arrive and you crave larger amounts of acid-forming grains, fats, and proteins, your body will already have a rich store of alkaline minerals. It's a natural, and effortless, way to eat seasonally and beautifully, and maximize your glow.

Beauty Science
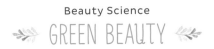
GREEN BEAUTY

You already know that eating leafy greens delivers a beauti-fying array of vitamins, minerals, and fiber that helps your skin to glow. But one recent study shows that those greens hold even more amazing benefits for your complexion—as well as your mood, weight, energy, and immunity—thanks to their hidden digestive benefits. Leafy greens (all kinds—from arugula and Swiss chard to kale and romaine) contain a unique sugar molecule that feeds and energizes the good, protective bacteria in the gut and helps it to proliferate, so much so that harmful bacteria finds it harder to take up residence. Consider your daily serving or three of greens to be extra insurance for a healthy gut and all of its many benefits for your beauty.

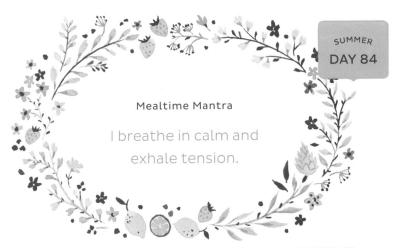

Mealtime Mantra

I breathe in calm and
exhale tension.

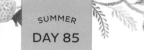

Kitchen Inspiration

LOW-SUGAR FRUIT

One key to blending up a smoothie that's truly beautifying is keeping the sugar—even natural sugar occurring in fruit—to a minimum. One of the reasons I don't recommend most juices as beauty drinks is their high-sugar, low-fiber profile. Sweetness may be welcome on our palates, but too much fruit juice negatively affects our blood sugar balance and, with it, our skin. Before you make your next smoothie, get to know the fruits with the lowest sugar content: lemons, limes, berries of all varieties (don't forget cranberries), green apples, grapefruit, and plums. Use one or two of these fruits in your smoothies to balance out the flavors of your veggies, and you'll have the foundation for a truly beauty-friendly beverage!

Time for Self-Love

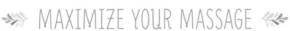 MAXIMIZE YOUR MASSAGE

Massage is one of my favorite self-care strategies, whether I'm kneading my own feet or getting a full-body rubdown from a pro. To extend the benefits, take a moment to debrief with the massage therapist *after* your next massage session. The advantage of chatting with the person who just had hands-on time with your muscles is some insider info about your trouble areas. You'll often receive feedback and suggestions that can help you correct issues in posture or movement—which will help you feel better ALL of the time!

Beauty Food Profile

EGGPLANT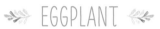

Eggplant will fill you up and load your system with beauty benefits, for only about 35 calories in a small bowlful. Eggplant is 90 percent water, contains lots of detoxifying fiber (be sure to keep the skin on to get all of that fiber), and has diuretic and mild laxative effects, so you won't bloat after eating and you may even lose some excess water weight. Take one look at the vibrant purple pigment of most eggplant skin (some varieties are white) and you'll guess correctly that it holds anti-aging beauty benefits. The anthocyanin pigments in the skin of eggplant rank extremely high for their antioxidant value and ability to nourish healthy collagen, and some evidence shows they may also protect against heart disease. Eggplant also contains a natural compound called chlorogenic acid that is thought to defend against cancer and fight free-radical damage, making it an important supporter of healthy aging.

EAT PRETTY FOOD	BEAUTIFYING COMPOUND	BEAUTY BENEFIT
Eggplant	Fiber	Supports healthy elimination

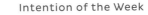

Intention of the Week

PLAY WITH NEW HERBS AND SPICES IN YOUR COOKING

Don't get stuck in a salt-and-pepper rut. Herbs and spices offer an incredibly concentrated treasure trove of free radical–neutralizing antioxidants to help us look and feel our best and age beautifully. This week, introduce unfamiliar flavors into your meals by adding herbs and spices in places where you would normally go without (say, in a smoothie or on top of toast with almond butter). And don't skimp—approach herbs and spices with a more-is-more attitude. If you're looking for a few new, and particularly beautifying, spice choices, go for turmeric, cardamom, and cumin (a few pinches of any of those stirred into warm nut milk is delicious, or add them by the teaspoonful into simple soups, stir-fries, and dressings). The classic staples parsley, basil, and thyme are bursting with properties that benefit your beauty as well. Use them, and discover an easy source of edible antioxidants.

Pretty Pairing

LEMON + SHRIMP

Why they're more beautiful together: Squeezing lemon juice over shrimp or marinating them in a citrus-based marinade before grilling or any other form of high-heat cooking has been shown to reduce the quantity of advanced glycation end products (compounds that speed up wrinkling and sagging in the skin) that naturally form during the cooking process by as much as 50 percent.

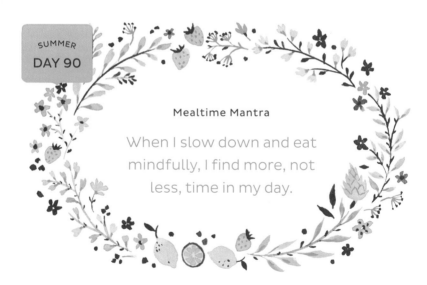

Mealtime Mantra

When I slow down and eat mindfully, I find more, not less, time in my day.

Beauty Science

❧ DIY DISHWASHING ❧

After cooking there's nothing more tempting than loading the dishwasher and letting an appliance do all the cleanup. But even if you have a dishwasher at the ready you may want to consider hand-washing your dishes now and then, especially if you tend to have allergic eczema, a common beauty woe. Turns out that little doses of microbes, like the ones that hang out on your dishes when they haven't been sanitized in a dishwasher's high-heat wash, are good for you. One recent study of over one thousand families found that only 23 percent of children in hand-dishwashing households had eczema, compared to 38 percent of children in dishwasher households. While you certainly don't need to shut down your dishwasher for good, this is more evidence that being a little less-than-clean can actually have beauty benefits. Double those benefits by using the extra time at the sink for self-reflection or deep breathing while you digest.

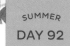

Kitchen Inspiration
STOCK FOODS THAT INTERRUPT THE STRESS CYCLE

If you've ever felt caught in a cycle of stress, know that probiotic-rich fermented foods can actually help to stop it. Constant stress from our busy lives disrupts and destroys the healthy bacteria populating our digestive system, making it even harder to manufacture the calming serotonin and happiness-inducing dopamine that are produced so heavily in our gut. More stress ensues! One way to interrupt the cycle and feed your body the beneficial bacteria it needs to stay on track is by consuming a steady intake of fermented foods—just a little every day is powerful for your beauty and health. Make fermented foods like miso, raw sauerkraut (see recipe on page 113), kimchi, and cultured vegetables one of the cornerstones of your beautifying kitchen and you'll support both physical and emotional beauty.

FAREWELL, SUMMER. BRING ON AUTUMN!

Having learned or put into practice more than ninety summertime Eat Pretty tips, do you feel radiant, energized, and ready to enter the busy, industrious autumn season? As autumn greets you, continue working on the skills you're developing to cook more intuitively, grace your meals with fresh herbs, spices, and whole food ingredients, and use more beautifying versions of traditional ingredients like grains and breads. Keep in mind what you've learned this summer: you've worked to redefine your workouts, prioritize mindfulness, and focus your attention on the aspects of your beauty that you love most, inside and out. Continue doing all of these things and you'll maintain your summer glow even as the days get shorter. Tomorrow autumn arrives, and with it comes a new set of needs and challenges for your beauty. If you continue to embrace the habits in the previous pages, you'll sail through the autumn season with confidence in your body and your beauty, and embrace each day as your best self. Turn the page and begin a new season of glow-boosting ideas.

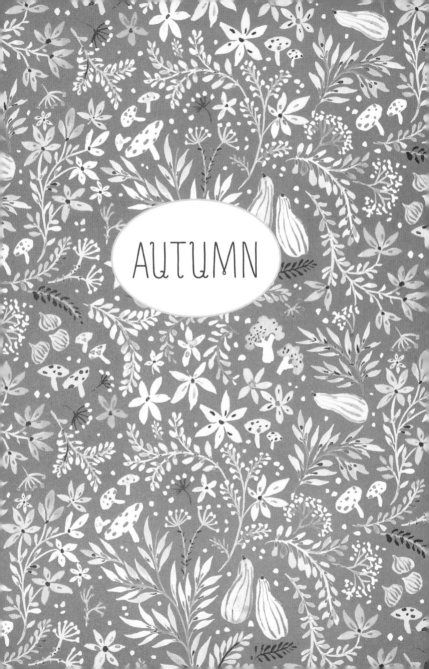

AUTUMN

Autumn is the season of gathering and grounding. Both concepts influence your energy and your beauty as you transition from summer to fall and strive for balance before the arrival of winter. It's easy to feel off-balance in your body and your skin this season, as temperatures, diets, and routines are likely to be in flux. Your skin-cell turnover slows, leaving your complexion more prone to breakouts and textural changes. Your skin and body need extra nourishment to allow for repair after the intense summer elements. Beyond the physical, packed work and social schedules during this season of industriousness push your self-care out of the picture if you're not mindful.

Use the daily entries in the pages ahead to experience a more beautiful autumn this year. You'll be encouraged to eat seasonally from the harvest of beautifying fall foods like pumpkin, squash, sweet potatoes, kale, and apples that fuel natural repair, detox, and glow. You'll aim to return to a more focused routine and work to pursue your passions this season, as doing what makes you happy also makes you glow. At the same time, you'll want to persevere in letting go of habits and foods that aren't supporting you. While you work diligently, you'll be reminded to develop ways to reward yourself that also deepen your beauty. You'll find many self-care ideas in the pages ahead, and in the Time for Self-Love entries throughout this book. At this busy, productive point in the year, your beautifying nutrition and self-care will create opportunities for nourishment, peace, and mindfulness that will keep your stress hormones in check and support your healthiest weight, energy, moods, and skin, as well as your immunity as cold and flu season arrives.

Above all, your goal is to treat yourself so well this season that you, your skin, and your body adjust effortlessly to the seasonal transition going on around you. And always be sure to listen to your body's needs, repeating the thoughts, intentions, and practices that leave you feeling radiant during the autumn season and every day.

Kitchen Inspiration

COOK YOUR GREENS

I enjoy introducing my clients to the benefits of raw greens because they're packed with beautifying properties, and they offer an easy, instant dose of nutrition and energy when blended into smoothies or eaten in salads. But cooked greens also offer major beauty benefits! In fact, some nutrients in your greens actually become more bioavailable when you heat them. Cooked greens may also be higher in available cancer-fighting phytochemicals and lower in oxalates that can interfere with calcium absorption. And many of the hearty greens widely available in the fall and winter—think kale, turnip greens, and collards—soften considerably when cooked, making them even more palatable. So, today, toss some greens in a sauté pan, add some to a soup, or wilt them into a stew. However you choose to eat them, you'll enjoy nutrient-dense, energizing food for your skin.

Intention of the Week

LET HEALTHY VANITY GUIDE YOUR CHOICES

Healthy vanity, you may recall from this book's introduction, is the desire to look and feel your best. Rather
than selfish or self-centered, it's a quality to be cele-
brated, because it helps you to stay on track with choices
that honor your best self. We all have some measure
of healthy vanity in us, but sometimes we need a little
practice to make it stronger and learn to confidently
trust our inner voice. This week, challenge yourself to
connect more closely with your own healthy vanity by
letting your desire to be your best self guide the day-
to-day decisions you make. You might choose to take a
walk after dinner instead of watching a movie, because it
helps you relax and digest. You might get up ten minutes
earlier to sit outside quietly and reflect before you have
to rush off to begin your day. Or you might invite your
friends to join you for lunch at a restaurant that serves
beauty-friendly dishes. At times, following your healthy
vanity will mean taking a break from influences like
family, friends, and media in order to make the choices
that help you look and feel your best. But deepening your
confidence in your ability to make beautifying choices for
yourself this week will serve you for decades to come.

Beauty Food Profile

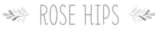 ROSE HIPS

Rose hips, which are the fruit of the rose plant, are prized for their incredibly high vitamin C levels—ounce for ounce, about eight times the vitamin C of oranges, though some varieties may contain up to fifty times more! They're also antioxidant-rich sources of several beautifying phytochemicals, including lycopene for UV defense. If you're wondering why you haven't seen rose hips sold as a snack at the grocery store, it's because the round, orange and red, berrylike fruits are a bit complicated to eat. The seeds of rose hips are inedible, so consuming them involves taking the time to scoop out their inner seeds and fibers. While you may want to experiment with collecting and deseeding rosehips to add a new beauty food to your repertoire, my favorite way to get their beauty benefits is to brew them as a tea, seeds and all, for a vitamin C–packed tonic.

EAT PRETTY FOOD	BEAUTIFYING COMPOUND	BEAUTY BENEFIT
Rose hips	Vitamin C	Powerful antioxidant defender

Time for Self-Love

GO UPSIDE DOWN

Downward dog, a beginner yoga pose, serves as a resting place and a point of balance for our bodies. Basic as it may be, simply spending more time in downward dog during your yoga practice, or at various times during the day, is a fabulous way to get the benefits of a more complicated yoga inversion (think headstand or scorpion)—including a boost in circulation, activation of the calming parasympathetic nervous system, and lymphatic drainage of your face, which in turn helps your skin glow—at any skill level. To enter downward dog pose, start on your hands and knees, wrists under your shoulders and knees under your hips. Tuck your toes and push up and back into a triangle shape. Your spine and legs should lengthen and straighten, your palms and feet should press into the floor, and your head should relax downward without hanging. The immediate flush you see after hanging out in downward dog will be temporary; the radiance in your skin will last even longer, especially if you make it a go-to pose to clear your head and intensify your glow.

Pretty Pairing

SPIRULINA + PUMPKIN SEEDS

Why they're more beautiful together: While mineral-rich spirulina alone adds a serving of complete protein to your smoothie, adding a handful of pumpkin seeds creates a protein source with optimal amino acid levels—and all twenty-two amino acids, including nine essential amino acids—that your body uses as the building blocks of your hair, skin, and nails.

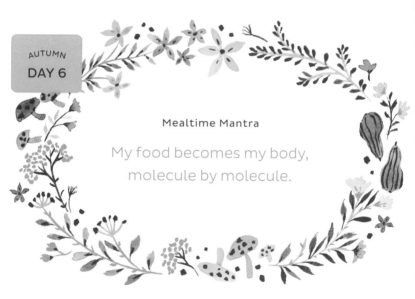

Mealtime Mantra

My food becomes my body,
molecule by molecule.

Living Your Best Life

HOW TO MAKE OPTIMAL FOOD COMBINATIONS

Ever munch on an apple right after lunch and find your stomach cramping up shortly afterward? Or finish a plate of eggs and hash browns only to feel uncomfortably bloated? Both of these are cases of food combining gone wrong. The science behind food combining—an approach to nutrition in which foods are intentionally combined for ideal digestion—looks at the rate at which foods are digested, and the varying enzymes required to do so optimally. Some people can digest just about any food combination with ease, while others get tripped up (and bloated) when they don't follow these basic food-combining rules: 1) Don't mix starches (like quinoa) and proteins (like wild salmon) in the same meal. To prevent inadvertently breaking this rule, decide ahead of time if your meal will be starch-based or protein-based. 2) Add as many veggies as you like, but reserve starchy veggies (sweet potatoes, corn, butternut squash, etc.) for your starch-based meals only. 3) Eat fruit by itself—not combined with a meal—either half an hour before or two hours after a meal. You needn't follow these rules all the time, but commit them to memory for days when you need a little extra digestive help.

Eat Pretty Recipe

SIP A SWEET FALL TREAT

CARAMEL APPLE SMOOTHIE

The flavor of this smoothie is reminiscent of a fall treat from childhood, the caramel apple. Unlike that sticky-sweet confection, however, my version tastes pleasingly sweet without added sugar (a major factor in aging and wrinkle-causing inflammation) and packs in skin-friendly nutrition, including complexion-smoothing beta-carotene, blemish-fighting zinc, and detoxifying apple pectin. Sprinkle in the optional maca root for a significant (yet stimulant-free) energy surge.

SERVES 1

1 cup [240 ml] unsweetened almond or hemp milk
½ cup [115 g] cooked pumpkin, canned or homemade
½ organic apple, cored (try a Macintosh or Honeycrisp)
1 Tbsp tahini
½ tsp ground maca root (optional)

Combine all of the ingredients in a high-powered blender and process until smooth. Serve immediately at room temperature.

Intention of the Week

UP YOUR VEGETABLE INTAKE

The vast majority of the population misses out on even the recommended eight to ten servings of fruits and vegetables each day. One serving is about a handful of veggies or greens or a piece of fruit, which means a recommended daily intake is about 2½ cups [about 350 to 430 g] of vegetables and two pieces of fruit. The thing is, even the recommended intake for veggies is seriously low if you're eating to look and feel your best! Introducing the Recommended Eat Pretty Allowance, which is the number of vegetable servings that feels right for your unique body—higher than what the rest of the population is eating. Every day this week, see how many servings of vegetables you can fit in, and see if you can you be consistent throughout the week. If calculating serving size makes you want to check out altogether, just remember this: the biggest section of your plate should always be vegetables. That portion size is win-win for your body and skin!

Time for Self-Love

LET GO WITH A LIST

Autumn may be a favorite season of many, but I know I'm not the only one who has trouble embracing it, as it means letting go of the summer season. I've found that one of the most effective ways to let go and move on from any loss—be it the warmth of summer or the passing of a loved one—is to put your thoughts in writing. For example, make a simple list of favorite memories. The act of pausing to write and reflect, regardless of whether or not you ever go back and reread your words, helps acknowledge your most meaningful moments. Sometimes looking back really is the best way to move ahead and embrace new beauty, with an open heart and mind.

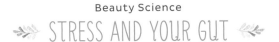

Beauty Science

STRESS AND YOUR GUT

One study observed that stress caused a decline in beneficial gut bacteria, while at the same time increasing possibly harmful bacteria and inflammation. Since our digestive health plays a major role in our outer beauty—including clear, glowing skin, a healthy weight, good moods, and immunity—it's essential to put daily stress-reducing practices into place in your life.

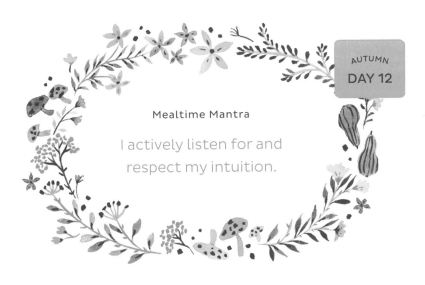

AUTUMN
DAY 12

Mealtime Mantra

I actively listen for and
respect my intuition.

Beauty Food Profile

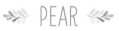 PEAR

In autumn, after the hot summer season, pears and apples arrive to cool and detoxify our bodies. The pectin fiber found in pears (especially concentrated in their skins) is a natural internal cleanser, known to support healthy weight loss and regular elimination. Pears are high in potassium, and their superfood skins are a good source of phytonutrients that boost antioxidants and reduce inflammation. When you can, choose red pears for skins that contain anti-aging anthocyanins that support skin elasticity as well.

EAT PRETTY FOOD	BEAUTIFYING COMPOUND	BEAUTY BENEFIT
Pear	Pectin fiber	Detoxifies and aids in weight loss

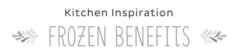

Kitchen Inspiration

FROZEN BENEFITS

One way to ensure that your body gets high levels of beauty nutrients at every meal is to simply eat foods that have greater nutritional value. While we often think of fresh produce as the most nutrient-dense option we have access to, frozen produce can actually have higher levels of nutrients than fresh, especially if fresh food travels long distances or sits in storage before arriving at your market. Carrots, apples, beets, and other produce are commonly stored, unfrozen, in a warehouse (or your fridge) for months, losing nutrition all the while. Frozen produce—which is often frozen immediately after being picked in a process that locks in its nutrients until you defrost or cook it—is an undervalued beauty food resource, inexpensive and incredibly convenient. Start hitting the frozen food aisle for budget-friendly frozen organic produce to use in your meals (the range of fruits and veggies available often make great smoothie, soup, and stir-fry ingredients) whenever you shop, and up the nutritional content of your meals.

Intention of the Week

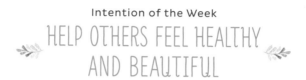

HELP OTHERS FEEL HEALTHY AND BEAUTIFUL

Remember that time you were having a terrible day and someone gave you an unexpected compliment? It changed your outlook. How about when you were recovering from the flu and your coworker dropped off a nourishing soup? It made you feel a little more like yourself again. We glow when we receive kindness from others, but consider that we may glow twice as much when we offer it. Research has shown that the most compassionate among us are more resilient to the effects of stress and have a greater level of well-being—qualities that nourish our inner (and therefore our outer) beauty. This week, I challenge you to do one thing each day to help someone else feel their best, whether that means complimenting their outfit or making them a green smoothie so they can start their day feeling healthy and energized. The more you spread love and wellness, the more readily it comes back into your life.

Beauty Science

THE DIET-ACNE LINK

One foundational study linking acne and diet suggests a direct relationship between the glycemic index of a person's diet—which represents how a specific food affects their blood sugar level—and the severity of acne. The study, done over a relatively short, twelve-week time period, showed that participants who ate a diet of 25 percent protein and 45 percent low glycemic carbs (think sweet potato, oats, raw nuts, beans, and legumes) decreased the number of their acne lesions as well as their weight, and increased their insulin sensitivity. To apply some of the study's findings to your life, focus on stabilizing your blood sugar with clean protein and healthy fats, and filling up your plate with low glycemic carbs. Skip high-glycemic foods like sweets and processed snacks. You may see a clearer complexion and a healthier weight overall in only a short time.

Living Your Best Life

HOW TO GROW YOUR OWN GARLIC

A single clove of garlic could be an anti-aging addition to pasta sauce—or the beginnings of a whole new head of garlic that you'll harvest in a few months' time. To grow fresh, antioxidant-rich garlic, break apart a head of good-quality garlic and plant each clove, pointy side up, in a sunny spot in the fall. Cover with mulch and watch for sprouts when spring arrives. Your garlic bulbs will be ready to harvest, dry, and cook by mid-summer.

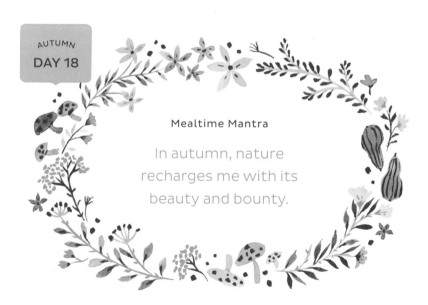

Mealtime Mantra

In autumn, nature
recharges me with its
beauty and bounty.

Time for Self-Love

CREATE AN END-OF-DAY TREAT

What do you look forward to at the end of your day? For many of us, our end-of-day treat is food-related, like an indulgent meal, dessert, or cocktail, built around ingredients that don't benefit our skin or our health. While indulging in healthy beauty foods instead is certainly a better alternative, it's important for the purposes of balance to offer your body and beauty treats that are not food-related. Settle on one or two ways to pamper yourself, unrelated to food, that you will look forward to throughout your day. You might crave a long soak in a fragrant bath, an evening walk, or time to read a good book or magazine. Don't let anything else cut into that end-of-day self-love time, and practice pampering yourself separately from your mealtimes.

Kitchen Inspiration
PRETTY (AND DELICIOUS) SALT SWAPS

Bloat never makes us feel beautiful. You've heard that skipping salt helps you avoid water retention, but it can be hard to avoid salt day to day. Fortunately, small doses of salt are healthy, especially unrefined salts like pink Himalayan salt and sea salt, which have their own potent natural mineral content. Still, overdoing any kind of salt will put you at risk for unwanted water retention. To avoid this, reach for beautifying (and delicious) salt swaps, like mineral-rich seaweed flakes such as dulse and kelp, which are often packaged in convenient shakers similar to a salt shaker. Their flavor is subtly salty and— don't worry—not fishy. Not only will you forego the excess water weight, you'll boost the beauty benefits of your meals, thanks to an extra dose of iodine, iron, and potassium, among other minerals, enzymes, and amino acids.

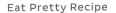

Eat Pretty Recipe

A BEAUTIFYING TAKE ON TAKEOUT

SHRIMP AND CAULIFLOWER FRIED "RICE"

This comfort-food recipe puts a beauty food spin on a classic Asian takeout meal: fried rice. Just as satisfying, it is incredibly skin-friendly, packed with protein (instead of simple carbs and unhealthy fats like you typically find in the original), and makes great leftovers.

SERVES 4

1 head cauliflower, roughly chopped and steamed
1 tsp coconut oil
1 organic onion, finely chopped
1 cup [170 g] fresh or frozen organic corn kernels
1 cup [155 g] shelled frozen edamame

½ lb [230 g] peeled fresh or thawed frozen shrimp
2 Tbsp low-sodium, wheat-free tamari
2 Tbsp toasted sesame oil
2 tsp rice vinegar
1 tsp maple syrup
2 scallions, finely chopped

Break apart the steamed cauliflower with a potato masher to form ricelike pieces. Set aside.

In a large skillet over medium heat, melt the coconut oil. Add the onion and cook until soft and golden, about 5 minutes. Add the corn, edamame, and shrimp and stir-fry until the shrimp turns pink throughout and curls, 3 to 5 minutes. Meanwhile, in a small bowl, whisk together the tamari, sesame oil, vinegar, and maple syrup. Add the riced cauliflower to the pan with the shrimp and vegetables and stir-fry until heated through. Add the sauce and scallions and stir until everything is well mixed and coated with the sauce. Serve immediately.

Intention of the Week

MINDFULLY FOCUS ON ONE TASK AT A TIME

One of the benefits of meditation is the heightened mental focus that comes from regularly tuning out the world. But if sitting down and being still for seated meditation seems daunting, consider that you can cultivate improved mental focus simply by keeping your multitasking to a minimum. Focusing on one task at a time, and returning your focus to that task whenever you get distracted, is a form of meditation. Research shows that multitasking all the time leaves us unable to concentrate, even when we're not working toward a goal. Our minds flit from one idea to the next and we have trouble establishing uninterrupted focus. On the other hand, concentrating on just one task at a time can reverse that trend and add increased focus, mindfulness, and peace to your days. Build mindfulness in your life this week by being present and focused on one thing at a time, whether you're at work or home. You'll retrain your mind and lower your stress at the same time.

Pretty Pairing
TURMERIC + BLACK PEPPER

Why they're more beautiful together: A few shakes of turmeric add important beauty benefits—including a reduction of inflammation and a dose of powerful antioxidants—to any meal thanks to its potent phytochemical curcumin. But if you remember to season with ground black pepper as well, you'll increase the amount of curcumin available to the body by a whopping 2000 percent. Even a pinch of black pepper does the trick, to more completely nourish your beauty and health.

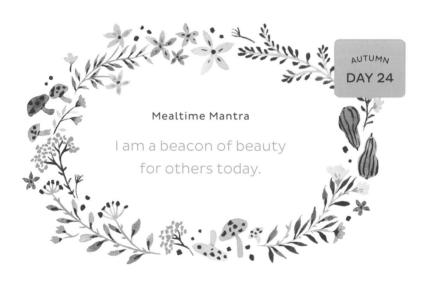

Mealtime Mantra

I am a beacon of beauty
for others today.

Time for Self-Love

GO ON A GRATITUDE WALK

When you walk, your thoughts can jump around as mindlessly as your feet stepping across the ground. Make your next walk more mindful by going on a "gratitude walk." Resist the urge to run through your to-do list or even people-watch. Instead, look around you, and inside yourself, and mentally note all of the things that you see and feel that fill you with joy and gratitude. Warm sun beating down on your face? A porch full of pumpkins? A violinist practicing in the park? These symbols of life can be beautifying when you notice them with gratitude. Gratitude has been shown to build happiness, reduce regret and other negative emotions (by increasing serotonin and dopamine in the brain), boost immunity, reduce inflammation, and support better beauty sleep—so go take a gratitude-filled walk today. (And while you're at it, you'll also be increasing the circulation of beautifying nutrition and detoxifying lymph in your body with every step.)

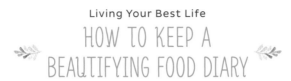

Living Your Best Life

HOW TO KEEP A BEAUTIFYING FOOD DIARY

Studies, including one extensive weight-loss study, show that recording the foods you eat in a diary can improve your weight-loss efforts by as much as double. But what happens when looking and feeling your best—not shedding a particular number of pounds—is your goal? Take a mind-body approach to journaling by noting your physical and mental states before and after you eat, in addition to your intake of foods. Focus less on recording portion sizes and more on using the journaling experience to help you assess your food-related feelings and physical and emotional reactions on a regular basis. (For a mind-body food diary that's built for this specific purpose, check out *Eat Pretty, Live Well.*)

Kitchen Inspiration

SKIN SUPERFOODS

When your skin looks lackluster, you could perk it up with a gently exfoliating and hydrating raw honey mask (one of my go-to topical treatments). But you'll get the best, longest-lasting results if you target your skin radiance from the inside, first and foremost. Start by reaching for the foods that give your skin glow-boosting nutrition, especially vitamins A and C, found in leafy greens, sweet potato, and bell peppers. If your digestion and elimination have been sluggish, or you've been indulging more than usual, grab extra fermented foods, plus lemon and lime for detox. And heighten the antioxidant value of all of your meals while reducing inflammation in your body by adding spices like turmeric, ginger, and garlic to your cooking. Then sit back, enjoy, and prepare to glow, with or without the topical treatment.

Beauty Food Profile

DELICATA SQUASH

One small serving (about a cupful) of cooked delicata squash has only twenty calories, yet it packs enough beta-carotene to deliver almost half of your recommended daily allowance for vitamin A, the beauty nutrient that balances sebum levels (preventing an over-oily or over-dry complexion) and aids in skin repair. During autumn, the season of renewal, squash like the pretty delicata are musts for a beauty-friendly plate. Each time you bite into a delicata squash, you're fueling your beauty with anti-aging vitamins C and B_6, as well as potassium, a nutrient that supports nervous function and boosts circulation to give your skin enviable natural radiance. I like to roast my delicata in coconut oil with a drizzle of maple syrup, sea salt, and antioxidant-packed cardamom spice.

EAT PRETTY FOOD	BEAUTIFYING COMPOUND	BEAUTY BENEFIT
Delicata squash	Potassium	Supports healthy nervous system function

Kitchen Inspiration

SMART AUTUMN SMOOTHIES

Leave the sweet smoothies of summer behind and blend up something to deeply satisfy you on a cool autumn day while fortifying your skin and body. This season, boost the beauty in your smoothies with these nutrient-dense sources of healthy fats: hemp seeds, for skin-calming and anti-inflammatory gamma-linolenic acid, zinc, and protein (opt for 1 to 2 Tbsp in a smoothie); an omega-3-rich oil blend, to reduce inflammation and nourish skin (try 1 Tbsp); and pumpkin seeds, for immunity- and beauty-boosting minerals and stress-calming benefits (try 1 to 4 Tbsp).

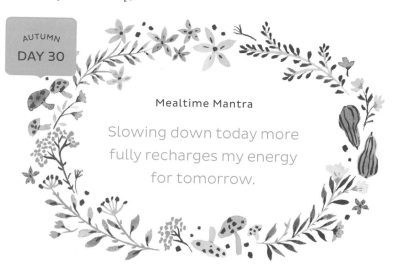

Mealtime Mantra

Slowing down today more fully recharges my energy for tomorrow.

Intention of the Week

ADD MORE FOOD-BASED OMEGA-3S TO YOUR DIET

Omega-3s. You've heard of them—now challenge yourself to find more ways to incorporate them into your diet. Omega-3s are healthy fats that support overall wellness by reducing inflammation, lowering blood pressure, supporting nervous function, and helping your body create new brain cells. But their benefits for beauty may be even more compelling. Omega-3s stabilize blood sugar (preventing wrinkle- and blemish-causing spikes); boost your mood; strengthen your skin barrier; assist in hormone balance; help produce healthy oil in your skin; nourish hair, nails, and eyes; and protect against UV damage. Although the recommended daily intake of omega-3s varies widely (ask your doctor for advice), it's possible, even easy, to get a significant amount of omega-3s from food: a handful of raw walnuts, a spoonful of ground flaxseed, or a palm-sized serving of wild salmon deliver a good dose. More omega-3 packed beauty foods to incorporate this week, and beyond: wild salmon, sardines, trout, mackerel, oysters, and halibut (all of which naturally contain EPA and DHA, two potent omega-3s); flaxseed, chia, hemp, and raw nuts, especially walnuts; and cauliflower and Brussels sprouts (which contain the alpha-linolenic acid that your body converts to EPA and DHA).

Time for Self-Love

SCALE DOWN

To build a happy, healthy relationship with your weight, say goodbye to the scale. Slide it under your bed or deep into your closet, and save the official weight calculations for the doctor's office. A scale gives you only one thing—a number; and for many, that number has the power to reduce a body to little more than a symbol of success or total failure. Instead of a daily weigh-in, measure your health in other ways. For example, assess your hunger level throughout the day, your digestive ability after a meal, your rate of breathing, or your food cravings. These nuanced measurements tell you so much more than your weight, which fluctuates by the day and hour. Developing new measurements can teach you to live not by the number that shows up when you step on the scale, but by your body's needs. In doing so, you'll build powerful self-awareness and hold yourself accountable for the way you feel and the choices you make all day long.

Eat Pretty Recipe

UN-SWEETEN THE HOLIDAYS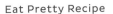

ANTIOXIDANT CRANBERRY-APPLE SAUCE

Cranberries are a powerhouse beauty berry, but a common preparation—sugary cranberry sauce—leaves our skin in an inflammatory slump. One cup [100 g] of fresh cranberries has 4 g of natural sugar and 50 calories (as well as flavonoids that support glowing skin). Compare that to traditional cranberry sauce, which has on average a whopping 88 g of sugar—almost a ½ cup [100 g] of pure added sugar—in the same serving! Today, enjoy these anti-aging berries raw in a smoothie, or make this tart, beautifying version of cranberry sauce instead.

SERVES 6

2 medium organic apples, cored and chopped into bite-sized chunks

3 cups [300 g] organic raw cranberries (about one 10-oz bag)

1¼ cups [300 ml] filtered water or freshly squeezed organic orange juice

1 tsp ground cinnamon

½ tsp ground ginger

In a saucepan over medium heat, combine the apples, cranberries, and water or orange juice. Bring to a boil and cook until the fruit begins to soften, about 3 minutes. Reduce the heat to maintain a simmer and cook, stirring frequently, until the cranberries pop and the apples are very tender, about 15 minutes, using the back of the spoon to mash the fruit to an even consistency. Remove from the heat and stir in the spices. Let cool and serve, or keep up to a week in the refrigerator.

Beauty Food Profile

BLACK PEPPER

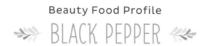

When we season our meals, we generally add salt more often than pepper. But pepper's ability to enhance the beauty benefits of your diet may convince you to use it more often. A phytochemical in black pepper called piperine (it's also the compound that makes you sneeze) enhances the body's ability to absorb essential beauty nutrients including beta-carotene, selenium, and B vitamins. Piperine in black pepper also increases the body's absorption of the anti-aging curcumin found in turmeric, so be sure to add black pepper to all of your turmeric dishes. As a bonus, black pepper has antibacterial properties and is known to reduce gas and support healthy digestion.

EAT PRETTY FOOD	BEAUTIFYING COMPOUND	BEAUTY BENEFIT
Black pepper	Piperine	Increases nutrient absorption

Beauty Science

NAP AWAY STRESS— AND WRINKLES

You know that a nap—particularly after a rough night's sleep—can restore your energy, but did you know it can also lower your levels of the stress hormone cortisol? One study of people who had had a terrible (two-hour) night of sleep found that their levels of cortisol lowered after a midday nap. Try a fifteen-minute snooze in the early afternoon to lower your own stress levels when you don't feel well rested. And, since elevated cortisol has been directly linked to signs of aging, you'll enjoy an anti-wrinkle beauty boost as well.

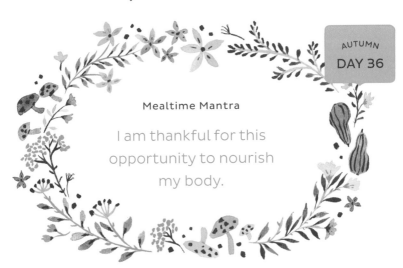

Mealtime Mantra

I am thankful for this opportunity to nourish my body.

Kitchen Inspiration

PEACEFUL PROBIOTICS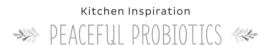

Ever notice that feeling calmer, more put together, and
better able to handle stress helps you feel more beautiful
as well? Turns out those feelings of serenity really do
originate deep down inside of you—in your gut, where
probiotic foods are particularly impactful. One study
found that, after four weeks of eating a probiotic-rich
variety of yogurt twice a day, participants were calmer
and less stressed in response to emotional triggers than
a control group that didn't get the probiotic foods. Brain
scans of the probiotic-eating participants showed that
they were less affected by the stressful stimuli, remind-
ing us of the often-overlooked link between gut health
and emotional well-being. The takeaway: probiotic-rich
fermented foods, from miso soup to raw sauerkraut to
kombucha and fermented pickles, can help you achieve
a calmer, more radiant you.

Intention of the Week

FIND NEW, BEAUTIFYING WAYS TO REWARD YOURSELF

When you were a kid, you may have been handed a lollipop for going to see the doctor, or ice cream after getting an A on a report card. It's no wonder that as adults our brains want an instantly gratifying sweet treat after we've accomplished something in our lives. But, looking at our reward systems from a beauty perspective, maybe we're not actually "treating" ourselves with ice cream and candy after all, since these Beauty Betrayer foods speed up aging, pack on the pounds, and make us more prone to breakouts, inflammation, and out-of-control blood sugar. This week, I challenge you to lay the groundwork for some new reward systems in your life. When you do something you're proud of, or you tackle a challenging situation with grace, you totally deserve a reward—just make it one that boosts your beauty and health as well. Try to turn the tendency for instant gratification into plans for bigger, more regular rewards, like a monthly massage, a new yoga outfit, or a concert you've been wanting to see—treats you'll find far sweeter than ice cream and candy.

Time for Self-Love

❧ USE A FACE OIL ❧

It's true that natural beauty products can be more expensive than many of the conventional brands you'll find at the drugstore, but my view is that you always get more potency and quality for the money you spend when you're buying natural. One of the most benefit-packed natural products you can buy is a facial oil blend, sometimes labeled as a serum, which works wonders for hydrating and protecting skin, and preserving youthful moisture as we age. Look for a facial oil with a blend of antioxidant-rich oils from plants like sea buckthorn, rose hips, avocado, jojoba, evening primrose, or pomegranate, with botanical extracts like calendula, chamomile, licorice, cranberry, or clary sage that target your skin's particular needs. An oil blend or serum from natural sources can absorb into skin even better than a moisturizer and lock in hydration longer, especially when you apply it to damp skin.

Kitchen Inspiration

BLOCK WRINKLES WITH RUTIN

News to know: one of the direct pathways to wrinkles, the accumulation of AGEs in the body, gets interrupted by a powerful phytochemical called rutin. Found in buckwheat, rooibos tea, mulberries, apples, figs, and citrus peels, this special beauty nutrient also has the deeply anti-aging ability to regenerate vitamin C as it goes through the process of neutralizing free radicals in the body—making it a must-have phytochemical in your beauty diet! Rutin also reduces inflammation and strengthens blood vessel walls, helping to prevent varicose veins. Add some crunchy buckwheat groats to your cereal today for an instant rutin boost.

Time for Self-Love
WORK IT OUT OUTDOORS

Get out of the gym or yoga studio today and create an unscripted workout outdoors. Walk on a beach, explore a nearby park, or rake leaves in your yard. Pay attention to the beauty you see and the senses you activate when you're surrounded by natural stimuli. You'll see the seasons changing before your eyes and take advantage of what may be one of the last few weeks of warmth before winter sets in.

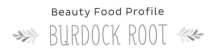

Beauty Food Profile

BURDOCK ROOT

Burdock root (which is literally the root of the burdock plant) may not be a familiar food, but its impressive benefits for detox, digestion, and elimination give it exciting beauty potential. Herbalists tout burdock for its ability to detox the liver and support kidney and blood health, both of which contribute to gorgeous skin. Some herbalists also recommend burdock as a powerful food for hair growth. Burdock root is packed with fiber that supports good bacteria in the intestines and is antibacterial, anti-inflammatory, and bursting with antioxidant value. It offers a wide range of beauty minerals like magnesium, iron, calcium, phosphorus, and potassium, and is a good source of B vitamins (especially B_6, a healthy hair and good-mood essential). Roast burdock root in soups and stews, eat it raw grated into salads, or juice it for a major beauty boost.

EAT PRETTY FOOD	BEAUTIFYING COMPOUND	BEAUTY BENEFIT
Burdock root	Vitamin B_6/pyridoxine	Supports healthy hair and good moods

Kitchen Inspiration
FIND YOUR TEA

Water will always be my number-one recommended beauty sip, but some teas come in at a close second, especially during the chilly months. Green, white, and rooibos teas get plenty of attention for their antioxidant values, but there's a lot to be said for the pleasure and comfort they deliver as well; choose the brew that sets off those happy signals in your brain while keeping the caffeine to a minimum. If you're looking for a new tea variety, try tulsi, a brew made from the holy basil plant that helps improve the body's response to stress. A tea you love can take the place of an evening cocktail or nightcap, and offer far greater benefits. For the most beautifying teas, look for organic varieties that don't contain added flavors.

Intention of the Week

TAKE A WALK ONCE A DAY AFTER A MEAL

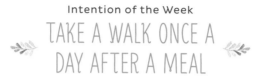

Curling up on the couch after eating may feel relaxing, but it's not always the most beautifying choice for your body—or your skin. Multiple studies have shown that walking, or doing any sort of light exercise, after a meal improves our blood sugar response, which affects the amount of insulin produced by the body, a major influence on skin radiance and aging. Walking just after a meal also has benefits for weight loss, as well as optimal digestion, as it increases circulation and promotes relaxation. Try a short, fifteen- to thirty-minute walk after a meal each day this week, and notice how it enhances your digestion and your skin.

Time for Self-Love

STEAM YOUR SKIN

In the time it takes to boil a pot of water, you can whip up a steam session to calm, cleanse, and deliver a fresh supply of nutrient-rich blood and oxygen to your skin. Oily and blemish-prone skin types can steam weekly, while dry and sensitive skin types should use this technique a little less often, around once a month.

To create a steam treatment, fill a large pot halfway with water and bring it to a boil. Carefully remove it from the heat, let it cool for one minute, and add a few drops of your favorite essential oils or a few sprigs of fresh herbs. Base your selection of oils or herbs on your favorite aromatherapy scent or your skin type. Rose and clary sage are wonderful astringents for blemish-prone skin, while chamomile and sandalwood naturally calm sensitive skin types, and juniper is antibacterial, anti-inflammatory, and detoxifying for your pores.

With your clean, makeup-free face positioned a few feet above the steaming water, drape a towel over your head to trap the warm air and breathe in deeply. Let the steam open your pores, increase your circulation, and induce sweating. When the steam begins to cool, splash your face with tepid water and pat dry. Apply your favorite natural toner and moisturizer. Since your pores have been opened and the outer layer of your skin is soft, your products are temporarily able to penetrate more deeply for even greater effectiveness.

Beauty Science
✏➤ BRIGHTEN YOUR WORLDVIEW ✏➤

Boosting your intake of carotenoid-rich veggies like kale, carrots, sweet potatoes, and spinach could positively impact your mindset, in addition to your skin. One scientific study found that its most optimistic participants had as much as 13 percent higher levels of carotenoids in their blood. Combine this finding with the skin-healing, complexion-smoothing benefits of carotenoids and there's no reason not to eat a few extra carrots today. You might see the world through rose-colored glasses tomorrow.

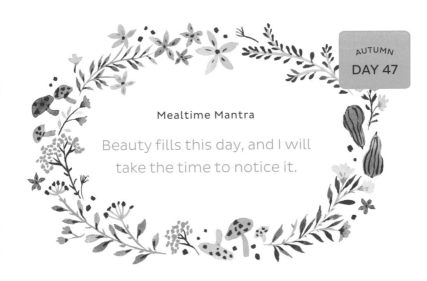

Mealtime Mantra

Beauty fills this day, and I will take the time to notice it.

Living Your Best Life

HOW TO PREP YOUR BODY FOR MEALTIME

Want to know one of the secret keys to a digestive system that keeps you energized and radiant? It's setting the stage for good digestion before every meal. This means drinking a glass of room temperature water about fifteen minutes before a meal to hydrate your digestive tract. It also means leaving the computer, smartphone, television, and stressful company out of the picture. And it means breathing deeply to lower stress and be present so you can make the healthiest food choices for your body. Try to check off this list—water, setting, breathing—before you sit down to every meal, and watch the change in the way you feel after you eat.

Eat Pretty Recipe

THE OTHER FALL FRUIT

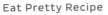

CINNAMON-PEAR CRUMBLE

Autumn is the season of apples, but there's another incredibly beautifying fall fruit waiting to nourish and detoxify you: the pear. This warm crumble is laced with cinnamon (to steady blood sugar) and ginger (for anti-inflammatory benefits), and topped with oats, buckwheat, and coconut to form a crisp layer filled with major nourishment for hair and skin alike.

SERVES 6 TO 8

4 large pears, cut into ½-in (12-mm) wedges	2½ tsp ground cinnamon
5 Tbsp [80 ml] unsweetened non-dairy milk	1 tsp ground ginger
	Pinch of ground cloves
4 Tbsp [55 g] organic grass-fed butter or coconut oil, melted	¼ tsp unrefined salt
	1 cup [85 g] gluten-free oats
1 Tbsp coconut sugar, plus ¼ cup [50 g]	½ cup [85 g] buckwheat groats
	½ cup [45 g] unsweetened coconut flakes

Preheat the oven to 350°F [180°C].

In a large bowl, toss the pears with 2 Tbsp of the milk, 2 Tbsp of the melted butter, 1 Tbsp of the sugar, 2 tsp of the cinnamon, the ginger, cloves, and ⅛ tsp of the salt. Pour into a 9- or 10-in [23- or 25-cm] pie plate. Set aside.

In a food processor, combine the oats, groats, and coconut flakes with the remaining 3 Tbsp milk and 2 Tbsp melted butter, the ¼ cup [50 g] sugar, and remaining ½ tsp cinnamon, and ⅛ tsp salt. Pulse until mixture begins to break down. Scatter the crumble evenly over the pears to form a crust. Bake until pears soften, about 50 minutes. Let cool slightly, then serve.

Kitchen Inspiration
❧ ROAST A PUMPKIN ❧

A pumpkin makes a lovely autumn decoration, but don't overlook its beauty nutrition benefits! To get the most from your pumpkin this season, use it as a display for a few weeks and then roast, purée, and freeze the nutrient-dense flesh for smoothies, soups, and baked goods all winter long. Cut your pumpkin in half, scoop out the seeds, and place cut-side down on a baking sheet greased with coconut oil. Roast until tender, and you'll have a major supply of this skin-nourishing beauty food. Even if you choose to carve your pumpkin, you'll be able to save the seeds, which you can roast and snack on for an excellent source of skin-clearing, immune-boosting zinc and the calming amino acid tryptophan.

Intention of the Week

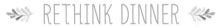 RETHINK DINNER

Dinner is an opportunity to nourish, recharge, and rest. But we often treat it like an end-of-day mini celebration in which we let loose and make choices that leave us feeling overfull, depleted of energy, or overindulgent. This week, rethink dinner! It doesn't need to be your biggest meal of the day, nor must it be meat-and-potatoes conventional. Try something easily digestible, like a simple soup, or a food packed with serotonin-boosting complex carbs like sweet potato, quinoa, or millet, which encourage restful sleep. Above all, approach this meal in a stress-free way, without the interruption of the television or computer, and eat only until you're satisfied, not overfull. It's your chance to nourish and pamper yourself with every bite.

Beauty Science

EAT CALM

Could the way you breathe affect your body's insulin response to the foods you eat? One recent study demonstrated that relaxed breathing significantly lowered the body's glycemic response, measured thirty minutes after a meal. The results suggest that a state of relaxation and calm after eating can change the way your body receives food, benefitting your skin, waistline, and the overall aging process.

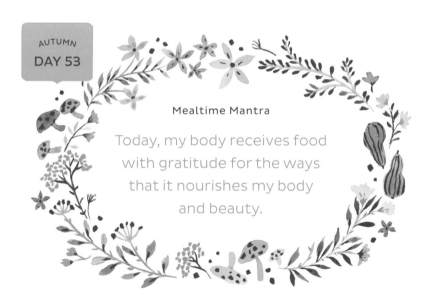

Mealtime Mantra

Today, my body receives food
with gratitude for the ways
that it nourishes my body
and beauty.

Beauty Food Profile

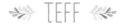 TEFF

This ancient staple is a model beautifying grain; it's gluten-free, high in beauty minerals and protein, and packed with resistant starch to keep you full and your blood sugar stable. One serving of cooked teff, about ¼ cup [60 g], contains 7 g of protein, the building block of your skin, hair, and nails, and a major dose of your daily magnesium, iron, calcium, B_6, and zinc. These minerals are key for a range of beautifying duties from strengthening immunity to nourishing healthy hair and strong nails. Teff makes a creamy, filling polenta or hot cereal, and its delicate grains can be ground into flour and used in protein-packed, beauty-friendly desserts.

EAT PRETTY FOOD	BEAUTIFYING COMPOUND	BEAUTY BENEFIT
Teff	Protein	Aids in cell growth and repair

Time for Self-Love

FEEL AWE-INSPIRED

When was the last time you stood in awe of a breathtaking vista, a staggeringly beautiful work of art, or a historic landmark? At that moment, according to one scientific study, you were directly supporting beauty, healthy aging, and immunity. In this study, positive emotions, especially awe, wonder, and amazement, correlated to lower levels of inflammatory markers in the body, suggesting reduced levels of inflammation and a healthier immune response overall for the participants. The takeaway: make time to seek out beauty that leaves you awe-inspired, both as a moment of self-care in your day and a path to long-term beauty and health benefits.

Kitchen Inspiration

STOCK UP ON INEXPENSIVE STAPLES

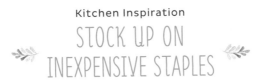

The next time you cringe at the price of hemp seeds or wild salmon (*So pricey! So worth it!*), remember to balance out your shopping bill with a few incredibly budget-friendly yet beauty nutrition–packed items as well. My top picks for beauty food staples that are gentle on your wallet are beans (even organic canned varieties are inexpensive, but dried beans are often even more affordable), millet, oats (although buying gluten-free can cost a bit more), and frozen organic vegetables. And overall, making any of your meals at home saves you major dough. That fresh-pressed juice or collard green wrap you paid top dollar for can power you up for a fraction of the price when you make it yourself.

Intention of the Week

EAT BEAUTY FOODS THAT ARE RICH IN BETA-CAROTENE

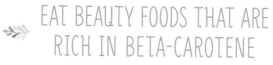

One of the most powerful nutrients to smooth and clear your skin, prevent and repair damage to your complexion, balance oil production, and give you a gorgeous glow from within is vitamin A, which the body converts from the famous phytochemical beta-carotene, among other sources. The great news about beta-carotene in autumn is that it's being delivered en masse inside the beauty foods of this season's harvest! To make sure you're getting your fill of this incredible opportunity for seasonal beauty nutrition, make room for beta carotene-rich beauty foods on your plate every day this week. You might choose carrots or butternut squash, pumpkin or sweet potato, or greens like kale, spinach, and even romaine lettuce. Pair them with a source of healthy fat (like coconut oil or olive oil) for optimal nutrient absorption.

Pretty Pairing
CINNAMON + MAPLE SYRUP

Why they're more beautiful together: Phytochemicals in antioxidant-rich cinnamon reduce the wrinkle-promoting blood sugar spike that results from eating sugars like maple syrup, a sugar source that also provides beauty minerals. Next time you sweeten your oatmeal or homemade cookies with maple syrup, don't forget to add a generous dash of ground cinnamon as well.

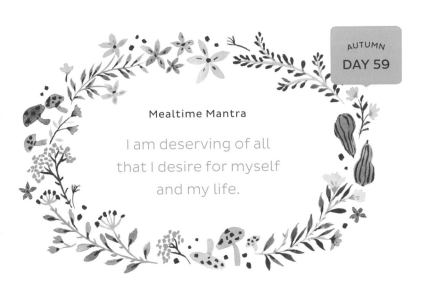

Mealtime Mantra

I am deserving of all
that I desire for myself
and my life.

Beauty Science

TRANSFORM YOUR BEAUTY WITH YOGA

The benefits that you get from regularly practicing yoga extend well beyond toned arms and increased flexibility. Practicing yoga also rewards you with dramatic boosts for your mind and healthy aging. Research supports that you can even transform your hormones and your body's stress response with this practice. One study found that once-weekly yoga practice (a ninety-minute session) over twelve weeks significantly lowered levels of oxidative stress and adrenaline, substantially raised levels of antioxidants (including the master antioxidant glutathione), increased serotonin, stimulated immune function, and benefitted overall hormone balance. Increasing your frequency of practice slightly, to three times per week, may be the sweet spot for yoga's greatest happiness benefits, finds another study. The message is clear: lifelong beauty, happiness, and yoga go hand in hand!

Time for Self-Love

STRENGTH-TRAIN YOUR RELAXATION MUSCLES

Liken your relaxation ability to a muscle in need of exercise. Just as weight-lifting repetitions work your muscles into top form, meditation, repeated again and again, develops the strength and overall ability of your body's relaxation response. Today, set aside ten minutes for a short meditation session. (You can set a timer to signal when you've completed your session, or go without.) Sit in a position that's comfortable to you; upright in a chair, hands in your lap, and feet on the floor is a good position to help keep you awake when you get super-relaxed. Close your eyes, start to breathe deeply and, as you do so, slow down your buzzing mind. The goal is to let your thoughts go for the next ten minutes. Focus only on your deep inhale through your nose, followed by a deep exhale through your nose or mouth. Whenever thoughts or noises distract you, simply let them go and return your focus to your breathing. Each time you return to your breath, think of it as one strength-training repetition (like one bicep curl). The more repetitions, the more your relaxation muscle gets toned and strong. Commit to meditation to strengthen your relaxation response the way you commit to workouts for your overall health. Only a few minutes a day make a big impact on your lifelong beauty from within.

Eat Pretty Recipe

A BEAUTIFYING BEGINNING

SPICED AUTUMN SWEET POTATO BITES

These eye-catching canapés are built on slices of skin-nourishing sweet potatoes and topped with raw walnuts, which are full of healthy fats. The natural sugars of grapes and pears mingle with fresh ginger in the spicy, cooked-fruit filling.

MAKES ABOUT 20 BITES

Melted coconut oil for brushing, plus ½ tsp

1 large, long organic sweet potato, scrubbed and cut into rounds about ½ in (12 mm) thick

Unrefined salt

1 cup [140 g] organic red grapes, quartered

1 ripe organic pear, cored and chopped

1 tsp peeled and finely grated fresh ginger

¼ cup [30 g] raw walnuts, chopped

Preheat the oven to 400°F [200°C]. Line a baking sheet with aluminum foil and brush with melted coconut oil.

Arrange the sweet potato slices on the prepared baking sheet and brush the tops with a little more melted coconut oil, then sprinkle lightly with salt. Bake for 20 minutes, or until tender and lightly browned.

In a sauté pan or skillet, heat the ½ tsp melted coconut oil over medium heat. Add the grapes, pear, and ginger and cook, stirring frequently, until the fruit is tender, about 10 minutes. Stir in a pinch of salt. Remove from the heat. Top each warm sweet potato round with a spoonful of the cooked fruit, then sprinkle with the chopped walnuts. Serve warm or at room temperature.

Beauty Food Profile

ROSEMARY

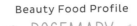
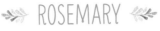

The herb rosemary is packed with antioxidant benefits that have been shown to dramatically reduce the quantity of aging compounds that form on animal proteins cooked at a high temperature, such as on a grill or under a broiler. And the anti-aging benefits don't stop there: rosemary's pungent oils lower the stress hormone cortisol when we breathe them in, and have been shown in several studies to boost memory. Rosemary is also a mood enhancer, making it a favorite natural scent used in spas and body-care products. Rosemary boosts circulation and its oils contain antibacterial properties that are traditional sources of immune support throughout cold and flu season.

EAT PRETTY FOOD	BEAUTIFYING COMPOUND	BEAUTY BENEFIT
Rosemary	Antioxidant oils	Defend against oxidative stress

Beauty Science
FOOD AND WRINKLES

One study looked at skin wrinkling in sun-exposed populations and found that the groups who ate a few specific categories of beauty foods showed the least amount of wrinkles. Exactly what were the beauty diets of these youthful-skinned individuals? They included a high intake of vegetables, legumes, and olive oil. A high intake of meat, dairy, and butter (all higher AGE foods) was associated with higher amounts of wrinkling. Mediterranean diet for the win!

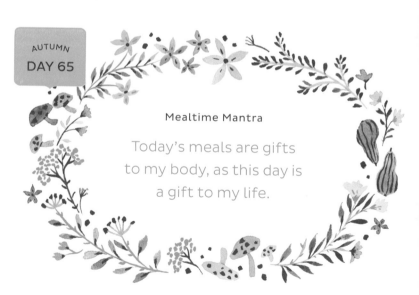

Mealtime Mantra

Today's meals are gifts
to my body, as this day is
a gift to my life.

Intention of the Week

EAT FERMENTED
FOODS EVERY DAY

To look and feel your best, it's essential to address the needs of your digestive system—the organs in your body that break down and assimilate food and process waste—making sure it is working optimally. Experts have discovered that much of what keeps your digestive system running smoothly are the trillions of bacteria that populate your body, called your microbiome. You not only want fewer of the potentially harmful or sickening bacteria (think E. coli and salmonella) hanging out in your digestive system, you want more of the beneficial, probiotic bacteria. One of the best ways to boost the healthy bacteria you carry around inside is to increase your intake of fermented foods, which offer a substantial content of good bacteria. Fermented foods, like raw sauerkraut, kimchi, brined pickles, miso, tempeh, kombucha, and kefir, develop this bacteria during the fermentation process. Since these foods have such powerful benefits, even a small serving, like a few forkfuls of raw sauerkraut, provides a substantial dose of probiotic bacteria. This week, I challenge you to get a serving of fermented foods into your diet every day, and watch the changes happen in your body and skin as you build up your healthy microbiome.

Living Your Best Life

HOW TO DETOX YOUR INDOOR AIR

Conventional, manufactured air fresheners are not the most beautiful route to refreshing your indoor space. Air fresheners, deodorizers, and scents for the home are typically loaded with synthetic fragrance and hidden phthalates, which are endocrine-disrupting chemicals that wreak havoc on your health and hormones. Instead of loading up on perfumed candles and room sprays that hide odors, clean your indoor air by opting for green plants that do the detox for you. A few plants that are best at filtering indoor pollutants are the peace lily, pothos, chrysanthemum, spider plant, English ivy, and philodendron, which typically require low light or little water. Choose varieties that will thrive in your unique living space and breathe deeply, enjoying the many benefits of bringing the outdoors in.

Time for Self-Love

MULTITASK WITH A MASK

My favorite way to treat myself while I'm doing chores, diving into research, or writing on a deadline is to apply a facial mask beforehand and enjoying its benefits while I task away. Knowing that I'm giving my skin a little love while I'm checking off a chore that I'd probably rather put off until tomorrow makes the job more bearable—even a little fun. Don't own a fancy face mask? Reach into your pantry and grab some honey. Plain, raw honey, applied to clean, slightly damp skin, is an affordable, highly effective face mask. Leave the honey on for at least twenty minutes (I've left it on for an hour while I got lost in work), then rinse it off with warm water and a soft, damp cloth. Honey draws moisture to your skin, loosens dead skin cells, heals blemishes and wards off future breakouts, and maintains the ideal pH range of your skin. And when your Cinderella duties are over, you can leave the house with the glowing skin of a princess.

Kitchen Inspiration

MAKE YOUR OWN VITAMIN D

Deficiencies in vitamin D—a vitamin we get naturally from the sun—abound for those of us who live in climates or maintain lifestyles that don't afford many opportunities for sun exposure—not to mention the limitations imposed by sunscreen, which blocks the formation of vitamin D in our skin. To ensure that we get our recommended daily allowance, we can take vitamin D supplements and buy foods that have been fortified with vitamin D (such as D-fortified non-dairy milks). We can also enjoy a secret dietary source of D—mushrooms. Mushrooms contain about 20 percent of your daily D needs—and get this: mushrooms that have been exposed to sunlight have even more, skyrocketing well above your recommended daily intake! For an additional, all-natural vitamin D boost in your mushrooms, leave them gills-up in sunlight—on a windowsill, for example—for several hours before eating them. The sun exposure increases their easily absorbable vitamin D content, which is a bonus for bone strength, immunity, and the skin's microbial defenses.

Beauty Science

DOES MILK DO YOUR SKIN GOOD?

While it's essential to recognize the need for a diet that best suits your unique body, there's substantial evidence that puts dairy into the category of foods to reduce or eliminate altogether—especially for the acne-prone. Several studies have found an association between milk consumption and acne, with one in particular showing that milk can cause a 10 to 20 percent increase in a key oil-producing hormone that contributes to acne breakouts. For clear skin, it may be best to abstain from dairy, or to use it as a condiment rather than a main part of your meal.

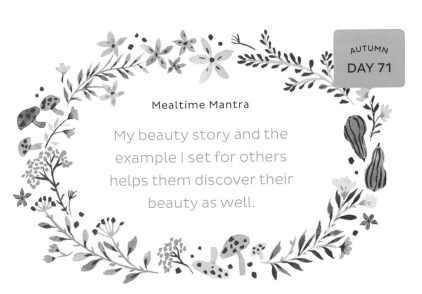

Mealtime Mantra

My beauty story and the example I set for others helps them discover their beauty as well.

Beauty Food Profile

PASTURED EGGS

If you believe that one egg is as good as another, prepare to be amazed. When you're faced with the choice of mass-produced, and always cheaper, conventional eggs versus more expensive eggs laid by pasture-raised hens, know that you'll get far more beauty nutrients for your money with the pastured option. One pastured egg (defined as an egg from a hen that has access to sunlight, outdoor space, and natural protein sources like bugs and worms) contains twice as much vitamin E and omega-3s as a conventional egg of the same size, plus a more favorable omega-6 to omega-3 ratio, which helps to keep inflammation at bay. One study also found that pastured eggs are seven times higher in beta-carotene than their conventional counterparts. Pastured eggs are also high in the beauty nutrients selenium for skin elasticity, B vitamins for overall skin, hair, nail, and nervous system health, lutein for eye health, and protein for building collagen, keratin, and elastin.

EAT PRETTY FOOD	BEAUTIFYING COMPOUND	BEAUTY BENEFIT
Pastured eggs	Protein	Aids in cell growth and repair

Intention of the Week

PLAN AHEAD FOR HEALTHFUL HOLIDAYS

As autumn nears its close, the joyous season of winter holidays is upon us. Too often, by the time we ring in the new year, we end up depleted, stressed, weighing more, and all-around regretful of our choices. Not this year! Start planning your holiday celebrations this week, with a focus on ways you can indulge while making choices that are more supportive of your long-term beauty and health. A few beauty-friendly options for sweet holiday treats include dark chocolate peppermint bark or hot cocoa sweetened with stevia, maple syrup, or raw honey; homemade cookie recipes made over with blackstrap molasses or coconut sugar (a lower-glycemic, 1-to-1 sub for white sugar); desserts that feature antioxidant-rich spices and almond or coconut flours; and creamy cashew cheesecake tarts with nut-based crusts. Get creative and create a sweet new holiday tradition for loving your body and beauty straight through the holiday season.

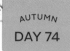

Kitchen Inspiration
RETHINK THOSE OFTEN-TOSSED ODDS AND ENDS

Did you ever consider that some of the food items you regularly throw away are hidden sources of beauty nutrition? Take broccoli stems, for example, which are one of my favorite smoothie add-ins for their sweet, mild taste and mega beauty nutrition from calcium and anti-inflammatory, hormone-balancing, detoxifying glucosinolates. Other often-tossed odds and ends that are nutrition-packed additions to smoothies are organic, unwaxed citrus peels, beet and turnip greens, outer cabbage leaves (as long as they're in good condition), apple skins, and the stems of herbs like parsley and mint and leafy greens like spinach and dandelion greens. Fill up your blender with these so-called scraps while you're chopping veggies for dinner, then top the blender off with some greens, lemon, berries, and water and blend them into a light, refreshing superfood smoothie with the beauty-boosting ingredients you almost sent out with the trash.

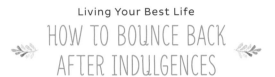

Living Your Best Life

HOW TO BOUNCE BACK AFTER INDULGENCES

It's happened before and it will happen again: you leave a party, wrap up a holiday weekend, or push away from the table after a restaurant meal feeling like "Whoa, that was fun, but I overdid it." So, where's the best place to go with your next meal? Tune into your body, which will no doubt be craving nourishing foods, and follow these guidelines:

1. Start with a green smoothie. Make it ultra-cleansing, using ingredients like dandelion greens, ginger, and lemon.
2. Opt for a light, nourishing meal like a bowl of soup.
3. Follow with a serving of fermented foods (or probiotics and vitamin supplements, if you take them).
4. Drink ginger and turmeric tea and go to sleep early.

The fiber-rich smoothie, the warm, easily digestible soup, and the tea support healthy digestion and elimination, while the greens and fermented foods restore nutrition and radiance to your skin. The extra hours of sleep you'll get from going to bed early help reset your body fully. The next day, expect to look and feel like yourself again.

Kitchen Inspiration
AFTERNOON SNACK TIME

Quick! It's four p.m. and you're starving. What do you eat for a beautifying snack that will keep your blood sugar stable and your body energized? Try these beauty nutrition–packed options:

- Raw trail mix
- Roasted chickpeas
- Hard-boiled pastured egg
- Apple with raw nut butter
- Chia pudding
- Pumpkin seeds
- Smoothie with avocado, berries, cinnamon, and coconut milk

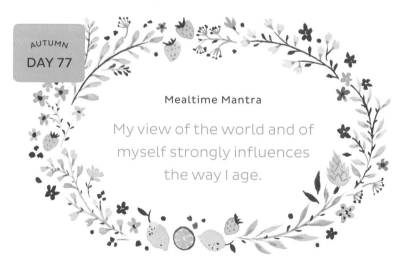

Mealtime Mantra

My view of the world and of myself strongly influences the way I age.

Time for Self-Love

LUNG LOVE FOR COLD-WEATHER WELLNESS

Runny nose? Scratchy throat? Colds really aren't very pretty. In the Eastern tradition, supporting the strength of your lungs helps ward off illness in the cold weather months. So what's the easiest practice for strengthening lung health? Deep breathing. Other traditional lung strengtheners include garlic, ginger, and turmeric (reach for them when you feel a cold coming on), as well as white foods like radishes, apples, mushrooms, and pears. When you're outside, keep your chest protected from cold air by wrapping up in a cozy scarf or zipping your coat all the way up. Lung vitality is closely linked to skin radiance as well, since it's one of the body's key organs of elimination. So look after your lungs to help keep your skin at its best.

Kitchen Inspiration

PRESERVE YOUR HERBS

As temperatures drop and the outdoor herb-growing season comes to a close, you may not be ready to part with your lineup of fresh, antioxidant-rich seasonings. These tactics can help you keep their benefits going as long as possible: 1) Bring your herbs indoors. Herbs like thyme, sage, and chives grow well indoors, in a sunny spot. 2) Make a pesto or dressing. A simple way to savor the concentrated flavor of fresh herbs in the winter is to make your own pesto or dressing and freeze small portions. Use olive oil as a base, and pack the recipe with a mix of basil, dill, parsley, and/or chives, blended in a food processor until creamy. 3) Freeze your herbs. Place clusters of whole or chopped herbs in the sections of an ice cube tray, cover with a little water or oil, and freeze. Pop these cubes into any recipe that calls for dried or fresh herbs. 4) Dry your herbs. Certain varieties like oregano, rosemary, and thyme are best for drying; you can crumble them into recipes for excellent flavor until growing season begins again.

Intention of the Week

MAKE MORE MEALS AT HOME

Cooking all your meals at home is just not always possible—or practical. Dining out is clearly a fun change of pace, and many restaurants offer beautifying dishes that you may not have the time, skill, or equipment to make at home. But home cooking certainly is beneficial to beauty, since meals prepared at home routinely have greater nutritional benefits and fewer Beauty Betrayers than restaurant and store-bought meals, which tend to be higher in unhealthy fats, processed ingredients, and empty calories. Beyond this major benefit of home-prepared meals, every time you cook at home you add to your knowledge of ways to nourish your beauty from the inside. So indulge when it feels right, but this week, save your basic, everyday meals for home prep, and savor the extra beauty nutrition on your plate.

Time for Self-Love

✤ HIKE FOR BEAUTY ✤

Here are three things you can do for enhanced health and beauty: Find a type of exercise that also lowers your stress. Spend more time in nature. Socialize with uplifting people. Want to check them all off at once? Go on a hiking excursion. The mind-body reset that comes from taking a long, vigorous walk in nature with a companion who makes you happy is the workout equivalent of a day at the spa. Studies have found that hikers are happier, and may experience an increase in antioxidant (read: anti-aging, beauty-supporting) capacity after hiking. Get out and see some beauty while you hike, and it could increase your own beautiful glow.

Beauty Science

GIVE AND GET IN RETURN

Getting a regular massage is a powerful self-care ritual for beauty and health. But several studies report that giving a massage has some of the same benefits as receiving, including reduced anxiety, lower levels of the stress hormone cortisol, and increased oxytocin, the feel-good hormone that rises in response to touch. Make time to help someone else relax, and you'll both feel a little more beautiful.

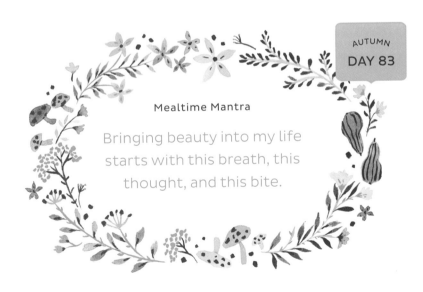

Mealtime Mantra

Bringing beauty into my life starts with this breath, this thought, and this bite.

Beauty Food Profile

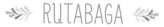

RUTABAGA

This white-and-purple–skinned brassica vegetable is a cross between a turnip and cabbage—and it offers the beauty benefits of both. Rutabaga, also called a swede, is high in vitamin C like cabbage, giving it major skin benefits. And like turnips, rutabagas are packed with glucosinolates that convert to the powerfully antioxidant phytochemical sulforphane in the body. Sulforaphane reduces inflammation, boosts anti-aging glutathione production, and can reduce skin redness and damage caused by UV exposure. Rutabaga is also a powerful antifungal food, important for fighting off unwanted yeast in the body, as well as a good source of potassium and a surprising source of calcium. Try it roasted or mashed, or even grated raw for subtly sweet, crunchy anti-aging benefits.

EAT PRETTY FOOD	BEAUTIFYING COMPOUND	BEAUTY BENEFIT
Rutabaga	Sulforaphane	Reduces redness and UV damage

Eat Pretty Recipe

A SIMPLE SKIN NOURISHER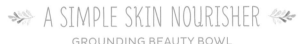

GROUNDING BEAUTY BOWL

During the autumn season, a simple grain bowl that includes nutrient-dense vegetables like sweet potatoes and broccoli is a meal that your body and beauty will crave. Topping this dish with raw, fermented sauerkraut adds a tangy crunch and further supports the health of your skin with probiotic benefits.

SERVES 4 TO 6

1 tsp coconut oil

2 leeks, white and tender green parts only, chopped

1 large organic sweet potato, scrubbed and cut into ¾-in [2-cm] dice

1 cup [240 ml] vegetable broth

1 large head organic broccoli, broken into florets

3 Tbsp olive oil

1 Tbsp red wine vinegar

1 tsp whole grain mustard

Unrefined salt and freshly ground black pepper

3 cups [345 g] cooked quinoa

About 1 cup [230 g] raw sauerkraut, or more to taste

In a large sauté pan or skillet, melt the coconut oil over medium heat. Add the leeks and sweet potato and cook until the leeks begin to soften, about 5 minutes. Add the broth and broccoli and stir to scrape up any browned bits from the pan. Cover the pan and cook until the sweet potatoes are tender, about 8 minutes longer. Remove from the heat.

In a small bowl, whisk together the olive oil, vinegar, mustard, and salt and pepper to taste. In a large serving bowl, combine the cooked vegetables, quinoa, and dressing. Spoon into bowls and top each portion with a scoop of sauerkraut. Serve immediately.

Living Your Best Life

HOW TO BUILD A BEAUTIFYING SELECTION OF CONDIMENTS

When you hear the word *condiments*, you probably think of staples like ketchup, mayonnaise, and relish. But there's a delightful variety of flavorful, beautifying condiments beyond these three. To build out your stash, start by adding healthy options that add instant flavor without loads of salt, sugar, gluten, or preservatives. Try low-sodium, wheat-free tamari or coconut aminos to add depth and umami flavor along with amino acids. And reach for antioxidant-rich hot sauce, or mustard made with beauty-friendly ingredients like turmeric and mustard seeds. Next, add condiments that pack a nutrient boost. Try nutritional yeast for B vitamins, sea vegetables for beauty minerals, and tahini or gomasio (page 70) for zinc and healthy fats. Then, look for condiments with antioxidant benefits like fresh herbs and spices. Finally, add fermented condiments that support digestion, like kimchi, raw sauerkraut, and apple cider vinegar (great in homemade dressings). Your meals just got a whole lot more flavorful—and beauty-friendly.

Intention of the Week
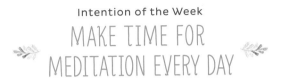
MAKE TIME FOR MEDITATION EVERY DAY

Meditation is often associated with spirituality, but many enjoy it as a non-spiritual health practice that is easily customizable to fit any lifestyle. Its many positive benefits have been documented in meditation studies, and its effects are truly beautifying to the body and mind. Experience its transformative effects for yourself. This week, take a few minutes every day to retreat to a place in your home that makes you feel safe and serene. Settle in, relax, and focus on the present moment while you breathe deeply. Let go of all other thoughts beyond the present moment and your inhales and exhales. Commit to this practice for a week (can you set aside ten minutes each day?), and try to keep going for cumulative beauty benefits!

Pretty Pairing

RAW WALNUTS + ORGANIC APPLES

Why they're more beautiful together: Not only do the protein and healthy fats packed into raw walnuts help keep your blood sugar steady while you munch on fructose-rich apples, one study found that a phytochemical in walnuts helps boost the action of quercetin, an antioxidant phytochemical in the skin of apples that blocks UV damage, reduces allergies, and fights cancer.

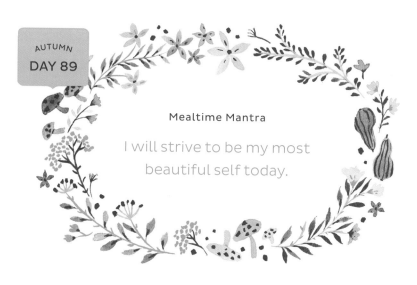

Mealtime Mantra

I will strive to be my most beautiful self today.

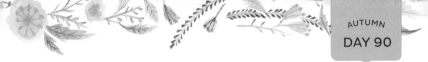

Beauty Food Profile
ROOIBOS TEA

Rooibos tea, also called red tea, isn't a true tea at all, since it comes from a legume instead of the traditional tea plant. But it still holds incredible beauty and health benefits. Rooibos tea is free of caffeine and low in tannins, so it won't interfere with mineral absorption in your body like some other teas. Rooibos has a slight natural sweetness and is packed with polyphenols including quercetin, rutin, and ferulic acid that give it a strong antioxidant value. Quercetin in particular is anti-allergy and has UVB protectant properties, anti-inflammatory effects on the skin and in the body, as well as anti-cancer effects. Rooibos contains the antioxidant enzyme superoxide dismutase that supports mitochondrial health, and has been shown to reverse some of the negative effects of stress on the body and regulate glutathione metabolism.

EAT PRETTY FOOD	BEAUTIFYING COMPOUND	BEAUTY BENEFIT
Rooibos tea	Quercetin	Defends against free-radical damage

Time for Self-Love

FIND THE "AAAH" IN ACUPUNCTURE

You know that natural endorphin high you get from just the right amount of exercise? It turns out that acupuncture—that incredibly powerful complementary therapy that involves the insertion of tiny needles into the skin to unblock the flow of energy, or qi, in the body—releases those endorphins as well. If you've ever left an acupuncture session with a giant grin, feeling lighter than air, you know it's true. Book a session today for a powerful balancing, uplifting effect. If you're an acupuncture newbie, know that the therapy has been found to be effective at treating an incredibly wide range of issues including chronic pain, nausea, digestive and emotional conditions, cancer treatment–related side effects, and skin conditions including acne, dermatitis, and loss of skin elasticity.

✽ SO LONG, AUTUMN. WELCOME, WINTER! ✾

With more than ninety autumn-inspired entries behind you, you should feel grounded and ready to embrace the restful, nourishing winter season. If you've channeled energy toward building beautifying practices into your routine over the past several months, you'll already see and feel major changes. If you're just getting started, feel excitement about what's to come! As the season shifts, maintain the powerful practices of eating an abundance of vegetables at every meal, incorporating fermented foods daily, and cooking some meals at home; these will serve you in any season. Be proud of how you've worked to redefine your reward systems, be more mindful day to day, and find deeper beauty in yourself by highlighting it in others. The beauty you've built in your body this season is far more than skin deep: it connects as much to your energy, positivity, and compassion as it does to your glowing skin and lustrous hair. Tomorrow, a new season brimming with fresh, beautifying ideas awaits—just turn the page. You can look forward to resting, nourishing, and reflecting during the winter season ahead, while recharging and preparing your body and your beauty for the arrival of spring.

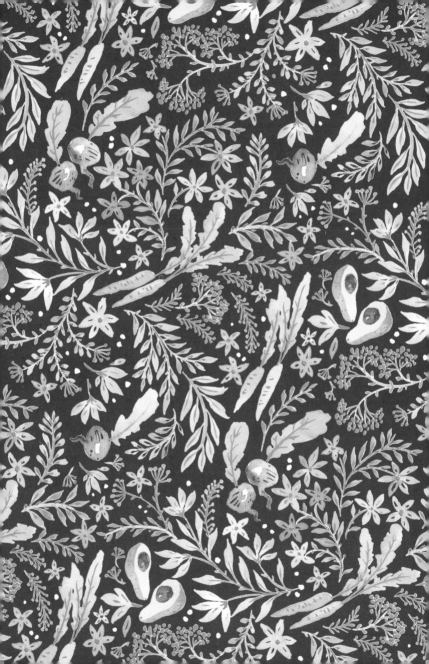

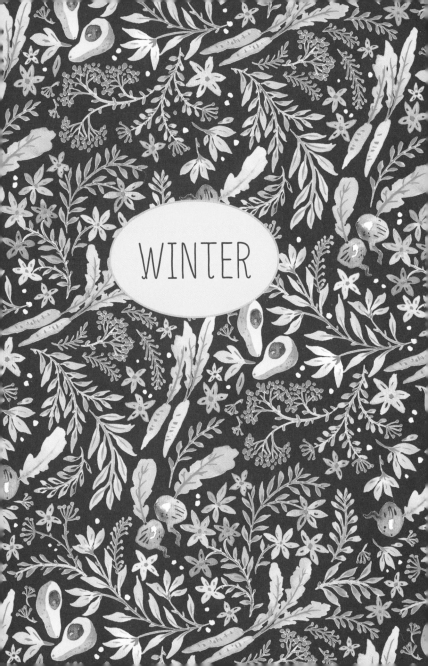

WINTER

Winter is the season of rest and rejuvenation for mind, body, and beauty. But since this season traditionally begins with joyful celebration and socialization, you'll need to make an extra effort to maintain a balance of healthy foods and habits that counter the all-too-common extremes of energy depletion, stress, and indulgence in foods that don't support your beauty during the holidays. As life quiets down later in the season, you'll want to embrace the long, cozy nights of winter by eating beautifying comfort foods, recharging, sleeping optimally, and pampering your body back into balance.

In the dozens of winter beauty entries that lie ahead of you, you'll see that while winter is a season to retreat, plan, and prepare for spring, it isn't merely a waiting period. Some of the most beautifying moments of the year take place during the winter, when there's time to surround yourself with loved ones who truly support you, practice self-care you might not otherwise have time for, and even experiment with some comforting new beauty foods in the kitchen. Self-love is a practice that deserves attention all year, but this winter you'll focus just a little more intently on developing the habits that best pamper and nourish your unique beauty and body. Of course, food is also at the core of winter beauty. Cold-weather beauty foods are major sources of pampering and nourishment, from the healthy fats that prevent dryness in your skin to the immune-boosting mushrooms, garlic, citrus, and spices that help ward off inflammation and illness, which you'll be encouraged to pack into your diet to look and feel your best all season. In the wintertime beauty entries ahead, you'll find permission to slow down, take time out, and deeply nourish with food and self-care, so that the arrival of spring will be even sweeter.

Closing one year and welcoming another during this season creates major opportunities for reflection and intention-setting that can lead you to make winter, rather unexpectedly, the most beautifying season of the year. Begin by turning the page and welcoming this chilly season with delicious food to nourish your beauty, inside and out.

Kitchen Inspiration

WHEN LESS IS MORE

Balanced meals that cover a variety of nutritional bases by including many different foods are a staple of a beautifying diet. But on those hectic days when you can't get in a balanced meal of diverse ingredients, remember that it's okay to simplify. How simple can you go and still be beauty-friendly? This winter, try a warm bowl of quinoa with a drizzle of olive oil and unrefined salt; sautéed greens with grass-fed organic butter and a clove or two of crushed garlic; an avocado with a sprinkle of spices; even a sweet potato with melted coconut oil will stand in for a meal when there's no time to make something elaborate—or nothing else in the kitchen! A hidden benefit of a pared-down plate every now and then is that your body has an easier time digesting the meal. Practice reaching for a nourishing, albeit simplified, plate when you're in a rush, rather than grabbing the processed meals and granola bars that are a common go-to.

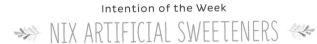

Intention of the Week

NIX ARTIFICIAL SWEETENERS

In the hierarchy of ingredients that nourish beauty from the inside out, artificial sweeteners are at the bottom of the barrel. Recent studies show that these fake sugars negatively alter gut bacteria and disrupt the body's ability to regulate blood sugar—two significant strikes against youthful skin. Artificial sweeteners are also known to cause water retention, headaches, weight gain, and sugar cravings. Even if you'd never pour one of those pastel-hued packets into your tea, you might not realize that there are artificial sweeteners hidden elsewhere in your life—from your chewing gum to your toothpaste. I challenge you to check labels, get rid of every last one, and make swaps where possible. For example, natural gum tastes just as minty as artificially sweetened gum—and without those sweeteners you'll be taking a big step toward lifelong beauty and health.

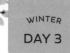
Beauty Food Profile

CINNAMON

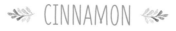

This warming spice is a winter favorite, though it deserves a prime spot in your spice rack year-round—especially if you have a sweet tooth. Adding cinnamon to foods stabilizes the resulting blood sugar spiking effect, so it's especially beneficial to sprinkle onto high-glycemic fruits or desserts. Cinnamon keeps us looking young by offering blood sugar balance, antioxidant powers (cinnamon extract in particular has been shown to increase antioxidant levels in the body by over 20 percent), as well as anti-inflammatory and immune boosts. Cinnamon is also high in the beauty mineral manganese, which defends our mitochondrial health. And there's another major benefit: one phytochemical found in cinnamon, a compound called cinnamic aldehyde, causes the release of protective enzymes in your cells. These enzymes reinforce the anti-aging power of antioxidants in your food, making their beauty benefits last even longer.

EAT PRETTY FOOD	BEAUTIFYING COMPOUND	BEAUTY BENEFIT
Cinnamon	Manganese	Defends mitochondria

Time for Self-Love

ENJOY A WINTER WARM-UP

For soothing, yet simple, support of healthy digestion (essential for radiant skin), get your hands on a hot-water bottle. This low-tech, inexpensive source of heat relaxes muscles and brings blood flow to your abdomen and digestive organs when you place it against your core after meals—exactly when and where you need it most for digestive support. I find the warmth of a hot-water bottle to be incredibly relaxing on winter nights after I've eaten a heavy meal, but I'll reach for mine in any season if I feel a hint of stomachache, bloating, or cramps. Try sitting with a freshly filled bottle on your abdomen for as little as fifteen minutes or up to an hour anytime you need extra digestive support. As a bonus, your hot-water bottle can help relax you into better beauty sleep when you use it during chilly nights.

Pretty Pairing

COCONUT KEFIR + GLUTEN-FREE OATS

Why they're more beautiful together: Coconut kefir, a creamy, probiotic-rich milk made from coconut, introduces beneficial bacteria into our digestive system. Once ingested, gluten-free oats (a prebiotic food known to help feed and sustain a healthy microbiome) convert into food that's used by our intestinal bacteria to survive and thrive. Pour a serving of coconut kefir on top of cold oats or warm (but never hot) oatmeal.

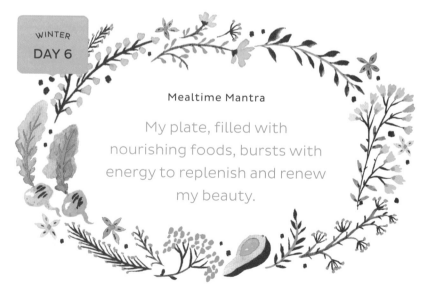

Mealtime Mantra

My plate, filled with nourishing foods, bursts with energy to replenish and renew my beauty.

Time for Self-Love

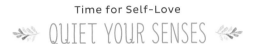 QUIET YOUR SENSES

Overstimulated much? The state of burnout that makes so many of us feel depleted of our natural radiance comes, in part, from our constant exposure to crowds, noise, music, media, and screens. While some of us thrive on this stimulation more than others, it's important for every one of us to set aside restorative time to simply *be*. Give your mind, body, and senses time to quiet down, the way you would on a walk through the woods, or during a meditation session; winter is the ideal season for this practice. Counteracting overstimulation in our lives helps us achieve deeper rest, and a more effective energy recharge that shows up in the way we look and feel! For a few easy, go-to quieting practices, enjoy a cup of tea, tasting each sip, or focus on nature by sitting in a park or even looking out your window at the clouds passing.

Eat Pretty Recipe

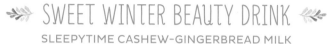

SWEET WINTER BEAUTY DRINK

SLEEPYTIME CASHEW-GINGERBREAD MILK

I love hot cocoa, but it's energizing, so not ideal to sip late at night just before you want to curl up in bed. The antioxidant-rich array of spices in this creamy drink support beautiful skin—and sweet dreams. Nutmeg is particularly beneficial for beauty sleep, so add a little extra if you need help settling down to bed.

SERVES 3

1 cup [120 g] raw cashews, soaked in water to cover for at least 4 hours or overnight, rinsed and drained
2½ cups [600 ml] purified water
2 pitted Medjool dates

4 tsp blackstrap molasses
2 tsp ground ginger
½ tsp ground cinnamon
⅛ tsp freshly grated nutmeg
Pinch of ground cloves

In a high-powered blender or food processor, combine the cashews, ½ cup [120 ml] of the water, and the dates. Process until no lumps remain, about 2 minutes, pausing frequently to scrape down the sides of the blender jar or work bowl.

Add the remaining 2 cups [480 ml] water, the molasses, ginger, cinnamon, nutmeg, and cloves and process until well blended. Transfer to a saucepan and heat gently over low heat until warm. Pour into mugs and serve immediately.

Intention of the Week

SEEK OUT THE COMPANY OF THOSE WHO SUPPORT YOUR HEALTH AND BEAUTY

Sabotage. We do it to ourselves, sometimes unwittingly, and we do it to others, perhaps with a little more consciousness, as suggested by a scientific study that found that we choose unhealthier foods when grocery shopping for others than when buying for ourselves—perhaps because we don't stop and think that they, too, might have health-related intentions they are trying to commit to. But there are clear exceptions to these tendencies. In your life, who are the people who support you without judgment, boost your self-confidence, keep you committed to your intentions, and respect the healthy choices you make for your beautiful life? Who are the ones who join along, reinforcing your healthy efforts? This week, seek out those lights in your life. Make a date to cook a beautifying dinner with a friend who shares your love of collard greens, or schedule time for a walk-and-talk with your sister who loves exercise like you do. When building your lifestyle of beauty, place those positive forces all around you!

Living Your Best Life

HOW TO SET THE TONE
FOR A BEAUTIFUL YEAR

As you anticipate, and celebrate, the arrival of the new year, pinpoint a single word that describes how you want to feel, instead of settling on a resolution or challenge for yourself. Take into account your current goals, the needs you want to fulfill, and the events or challenges you foresee in the year ahead. In the past, some words that I've chosen have been: relaxed (when I was facing major life stress), open (when I wanted to attract new energy and opportunity), and vital (when I wanted to create, move, and take action). Write this word in a place where you'll see it often, and let it weave its way through your year. Whenever you're facing a big decision, or wondering how to fill a free afternoon, let this word be your guide. Try to evoke this feeling day after day, and let it bring you exactly what you need.

Beauty Science
SLEEP TO STAY WELL

Sleep is free anti-aging, and it's also a free immune boost. One recent study found that participants who slept less than six hours were more than four times more likely to catch a cold virus than those who slept seven hours or more. When it comes to looking and feeling beautiful this winter, staying cold-free is key. Use this season of rest to renew your skin and boost your immunity with full nights of sleep.

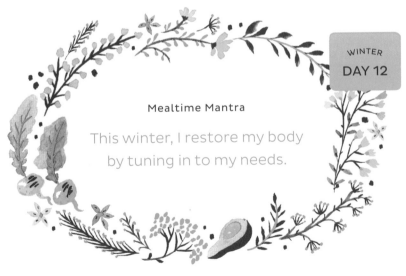

Mealtime Mantra

This winter, I restore my body by tuning in to my needs.

Kitchen Inspiration

CITRUS PEELS FOR CELLULITE PREVENTION

Citrus peels and piths (the bitter white stuff on the underside of the peel) offer not-to-be-missed support for your skin and blood vessels. Several citrus bioflavonoids strengthen blood vessels and microcirculation to help prevent varicose veins and swelling of the legs and ankles; provide anti-inflammatory benefits; and support the healthy movement of detoxifying lymph throughout the body, which in turn helps prevent cellulite. Since you probably won't want to snack on bitter citrus peels (and the sugar content of candied peels negates their beauty benefits), sneak them into your diet in other ways. Try blending a few strips of organic lemon peel (with the pith intact) into your smoothies for a burst of citrus flavor without detectable bitterness. And grating lemon, lime, orange, or even grapefruit zest into dressings and over salads and sweets is another tasty way to support your skin from within, by using an ingredient you might otherwise send down the garbage disposal. Make sure your citrus fruits are unwaxed and organic, and you'll soon be sipping your way to cellulite prevention from the inside out.

Beauty Food Profile

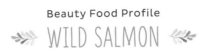

WILD SALMON

The concentrated omega-3 content of wild salmon makes it a fabulous protein source for beauty. Omega-3s in wild salmon are strongly anti-inflammatory, and may improve acne and eczema and defend against sun damage. The protein in wild salmon (about 23 g in a 3-oz/85-g serving) stabilizes blood sugar and satisfies you, even as it delivers building blocks for your skin, hair, and nails. Beyond its healthy fats and protein, wild salmon is an excellent source of selenium for skin elasticity, as well as several B vitamins including B_3, B_6, and B_{12}. Wild salmon also contains astaxanthin, a super-potent antioxidant pigment that gives salmon its pink color and may reduce DNA damage in our bodies as well as protect against sunburn. For the best quality salmon, choose wild over farm-raised, since farmed salmon may contain unwanted colors and antibiotics.

EAT PRETTY FOOD	BEAUTIFYING COMPOUND	BEAUTY BENEFIT
Wild salmon	Omega-3s	Reduce inflammation and protect skin from UV damage

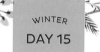

Time for Self-Love

CONSCIOUSLY RELAX

Whether you regularly fall asleep the second you climb under the covers or lie awake until you manage to drift to dreamland, there may be a better way to ease into bedtime. Use the moments between the time your head hits the pillow and you start snoozing to consciously relax. The practice, called progressive relaxation, is simple. After you lie down, close your eyes and mentally connect with each part of your body, starting with your toes and moving up to your head. Purposefully tense and relax each area, from feet to ankles to thighs, stomach to arms and shoulders, working to release areas of stress and tension. If you find a spot that feels clenched, move it, massage it, or otherwise release that stress to get yourself into an optimal sleep state. This practice works even better than counting sheep to get you prepped for beauty rest!

Intention of the Week

OVERHAUL YOUR KITCHEN OILS

You've heard of healthy fats. But are you familiar with *beautifying* fats? Some of the most widely used cooking oils, like canola and vegetable oils, are typically chemically extracted, highly refined, and bleached, which reduces their beauty benefits considerably. As a result, these oils become inflammatory in the body, and that inflammation is a factor in wrinkling, premature aging, and red, sensitive skin. Toss out those old oils and switch to skin-friendly coconut oil as your all-purpose, high-heat cooking oil. This fat, which is anti-inflammatory, is preferable for grilling, stir-frying, and roasting; it also metabolizes quickly for energy and nourishes healthy cell membranes and gorgeous skin. Other beautifying fats are cold-pressed extra-virgin olive, flax, avocado, and hemp oils, which are great for drizzling over food and making dressings. These contain beneficial mono- and polyunsaturated fats that fare better at low temps. Hemp oil in particular has an ideal 3:1 ratio of omega-3s to omega-6s, plus skin-friendly gamma-linolenic acid. Continue your exploration of beautifying fats by trying sesame oil, ghee, or organic grass-fed butter—all fabulous fats for skin and beauty that deserve a place in your pantry as well.

Time for Self-Love

SOURCE SAFE LIPSTICK

Lipstick can instantly upgrade your look—but not if it's simultaneously dosing your body with contaminants like lead. Since you can't help ingesting small amounts of lipstick every time you apply it (which can add up to several pounds over a lifetime), source your lipstick from one of the many organic or nontoxic brands out there, one with products that have been tested and proven to be free of lead and other heavy metals. With a truly safe lipstick in your beauty routine, you won't hesitate to go ahead and apply another coat.

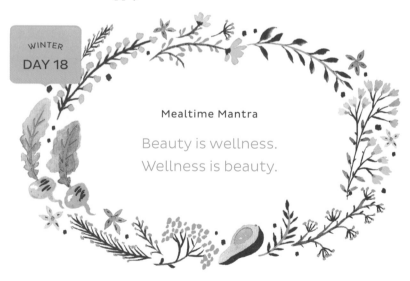

Mealtime Mantra

Beauty is wellness.
Wellness is beauty.

Kitchen Inspiration

MAXIMIZE THE BENEFITS OF MAGNESIUM

Want proof that just one nutrient can make or break your beauty regimen? Low magnesium levels alone can hasten aging by increasing free radicals and making your cells more susceptible to damage. Of course magnesium is crucial for more than just age defense; it's a calming mineral and a powerful detoxifier. Magnesium increases mood-lifting serotonin and relaxes muscles, making it an essential nutrient for the chronically stressed. Some of my favorite magnesium-rich beauty foods are leafy greens, cashews, quinoa, and pumpkin seeds, although you can also supplement effectively with a powdered magnesium drink or a soak in a bath containing Epsom salts. This last method is an ideal daily calming ritual, and it's one of my top picks for lowering stress hormones over time. Sprinkle a large scoop of Epsom salts in warm bath water and soak for at least twenty minutes for optimal magnesium absorption.

Living Your Best Life

HOW TO CREATE A SLEEP SANCTUARY

You know that sleep is a deeply restorative action for your beauty and body, and that winter is the season to prioritize that restoration. But did you also know that your skin cells respond to certain triggers that put them into rejuvenation mode? Turning your bedroom in to a beauty sleep sanctuary can help you sleep deeper and recharge better. The first thing on your to-do list is to remove your TV from your bedroom. While you're at it, remove all of your devices, since they emit a type of light that disrupts your body's melatonin production, sleep, and even mood. Set the thermostat to a comfortable temperature between 55° and 75°F [13° and 24°C]. Plug in a scent-diffusing humidifier to keep your skin dewy and add a few drops of your favorite calming essential oil like lavender, sandalwood, or vetiver. If outside sounds distract you, add some white noise, like the sound of ocean waves or light rain. For long-term health and beauty, consider a mattress built from nontoxic materials like natural wood, and organic fabrics and fillers. (So many cumulative hours are spent in close contact with your mattress, and undesirable chemicals are applied heavily to many of the materials in conventional mattresses.) Overall, keep your bedroom uncluttered and unspoiled, and you'll have a smoother transition to sleep, wake with deeper glow, and look forward to your precious pillow time.

Intention of the Week

EXPLORE A SECRET IMMUNITY FOOD—MUSHROOMS

You've heard that garlic is a prime cold-chaser, and you know that vitamin C-packed citrus may help you stave off sniffles. But to take your winter wellness to the next level, tap into the powerful immunity and beauty boosts offered by mushrooms. Not only do exotic mushroom varieties like shiitakes add umami flavor to your cooking, many have been shown to be antiviral, anti-inflammatory, and healing to those with compromised immunity. Mushrooms rank high in the superfoods that make beauty magic: they contain selenium for skin elasticity, B vitamins, even the important-for-immunity vitamin D. Both white button mushrooms and portobellos have health benefits, but how often do you cook with shiitake, oyster, hen-of-the-woods, enoki, and other more exotic mushroom types? Challenge yourself to buy at least two different kinds of edible mushrooms and try them in your meals this week. Sauté them in coconut oil and garlic to top a salad or polenta; scramble them up with pastured eggs (see the recipe on page 29). For more mushroom benefits, try one of the growing number of medicinal mushroom powders that can be added to smoothies; you'll find varieties like *Cordyceps*, Lion's Mane, and reishi that offer a broad spectrum of health and beauty benefits, even in small amounts.

Eat Pretty Recipe

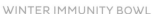

EATING FOR WINTER WELLNESS

WINTER IMMUNITY BOWL

A winter diet that supports beauty and wellness benefits strongly from two things: less sugar (which lowers your ability to fight off illness) and more immune-boosting superfoods, like garlic, ginger, turmeric, and mushrooms. This recipe has them all if you pair it with Tangy Turmeric-Lemon Dressing (page 311). This ultra-simple meal is ideal for chasing away a cold—or even preventing one—while reducing seasonal inflammation in your skin.

SERVES 2

1 cup [240 ml] vegetable broth
½ cup [120 ml] purified water
¾ cup [130 g] buckwheat groats, rinsed and drained
1 tsp coconut oil

2 portobello mushroom caps, stems and gills removed, cut into ½-in (12-mm) slices
2 cloves garlic, minced
½ lb [230 g] Brussels sprouts, halved

In a small saucepan over medium-high heat, combine the broth and water and bring to a boil. Add the buckwheat, reduce the heat to medium-low, and simmer until tender, about 15 minutes. Remove from the heat, drain any remaining liquid, and set aside. While the buckwheat is cooking, melt the coconut oil in a sauté pan or skillet over medium heat. Add the mushrooms, garlic, and Brussels sprouts and cook, stirring frequently, until the mushrooms are soft and nicely browned and the sprouts are tender, about 8 minutes. Divide the buckwheat between two bowls and top with the vegetables and your favorite dressing (see recipe introduction). Serve immediately.

Pretty Pairing
ROOIBOS TEA + DARK CHOCOLATE

Why they're more beautiful together: Skip the cookie and pair your cozy cup of rooibos tea with a square or two of dark chocolate to support beautiful circulation, an essential for gorgeous skin and energy. The beauty magic is in the phytochemical combination of quercetin, found in rooibos tea, and catechins, abundant in dark chocolate, which work together to thin blood and strengthen your cardiovascular health.

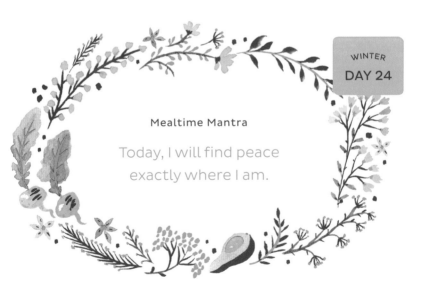

Mealtime Mantra

Today, I will find peace
exactly where I am.

Beauty Food Profile

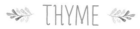

THYME

Rich in savory flavor, antioxidants, and anti-inflammatory properties, thyme is a staple herb in your beauty kitchen. Thyme's most powerful component, thymol, is anti-bacterial, antiviral (you'll find thyme used in oral products like mouthwash), and supportive of digestive health, since it kills off unwanted bacteria like *H. pylori*. In studies, thyme oil has shown the ability to increase the concentration of omega-3s in the body, possibly making your omega-3-rich foods more effective. Another study found that thyme oil slowed age-related reductions in an enzyme called superoxide dismutase that supports mito-chondrial health, as well as the strong antioxidant gluta-thione. Try consuming your thyme fresh (it's a hearty, easy-to-grow herb) for the most potent antioxidant benefits.

EAT PRETTY FOOD	BEAUTIFYING COMPOUND	BEAUTY BENEFIT
Thyme	Thymol	Destroys unwanted bacteria

Kitchen Inspiration

MAKE YOUR OWN NON-DAIRY MILKS

Beyond their beautifying fats and creamy texture, non-dairy milks make ideal replacements for those allergic to dairy or seeking to avoid conventional milk's potential to spur inflammation and breakouts. While it's incredibly convenient to buy non-dairy milk at the grocery store, if you're not careful, you'll find that there can be extra ingredients (like flavors, thickeners, preservatives, and sweeteners) added to what you thought was just a basic product. If you have the time, initiative, or need some creamy, dairy-free milk in a pinch, it helps to know how to make your own. You'll generally want to use a high-powered blender or food processor to blend one part soaked nuts or seeds with two parts filtered water. Add a pinch of salt, vanilla, cinnamon, a few dates for sweetness, or any other flavorings you like. Depending on the strength of your machine, or how much you mind sediment, you may also want to strain the final product through cheesecloth or a fine-mesh strainer. For a creamy, non-dairy milk that doesn't involve straining or soaking, blend 1 cup [160 g] shelled hemp seeds with 2 cups [480 ml] water. The final product is packed with skin-nourishing gamma-linolenic acid, protein, iron, and zinc. You can also blend up 1 Tbsp nut butter with 1 cup [240 ml] water to make non-dairy milk in a hurry.

Kitchen Inspiration

USE YOUR SENSES AT MEALTIME

Turning mealtime into a pampering experience for our bodies comes naturally if we pay close attention to the beauty of what we're eating. But on busy days, I'm guilty of rushing through a meal so quickly that I don't taste a thing. That's when I remind myself to slow down, as you can do too, using a simple exercise in mindful eating. Pick one food, whether it's the first bite of the meal you're about to eat, or a single item like a chocolate truffle or strawberry, and practice using your senses to savor it. Pick up the food with your utensil or fingers, look at its colors and texture, and feel its weight. Breathe in its aroma as you lift it to your mouth in preparation for a bite. Open your mouth to receive it, bite down, and taste the first sensation on your tongue. Does its flavor change as you chew? Chew longer than you normally would before swallowing. Do any tastes linger in your mouth? While you may not be able to experience each bite this way, returning to this practice now and then is a wonderful reminder to be mindful and present at every meal.

Intention of the Week

REDUCE YOUR CAFFEINE INTAKE
AND TRY BEAUTY-FRIENDLY SWAPS
FOR YOUR DAILY BREW

Like you, I've heard many confusing and conflicting reports about the benefits and/or drawbacks of coffee. It seems like everyone has a different message about coffee these days. Like all foods, coffee affects each of us a little differently. But here's my take: if your goal is radiant skin and overall beauty, then it's time to break up with this caffeinated drink. Beauty is closely tied to hormonal health, and coffee introduces several obstacles to hormonal balance, as it overstimulates the adrenal glands, boosts our cortisol production, and negatively affects our blood sugar. It also interferes with our absorption of beauty minerals, acidifies the body, and often disrupts beauty sleep. In light of this, I challenge you to dial back your coffee intake this week, especially if hormone balance is a top concern of yours. To make this easier, and more sustainable, first think about why you like it. Is it the energy buzz? Green tea makes a great energizing swap, with added beauty benefits. Is it the roasty flavor? Roasted dandelion tea is a tasty alternative (my favorite brand comes in a powdered form that you add to water). Remember that when you support blood sugar balance and hormonal balance, you'll begin to discover more energy naturally without stimulants.

Time for Self-Love

EVERYTHING OLD IS NEW AGAIN

Today, challenge the "younger is better" mindset. Rather than living with the goal of avoiding aging (at which we're doomed to fail), focus on all of the beauty you will get to experience on your life's journey. Think as well about the powerful tools you're developing that have the potential to fill your years with health, beauty, energy, and self-love. When you resolve to seek beauty in each day of your life, you glow in a way that overshadows every line, wrinkle, and grey hair.

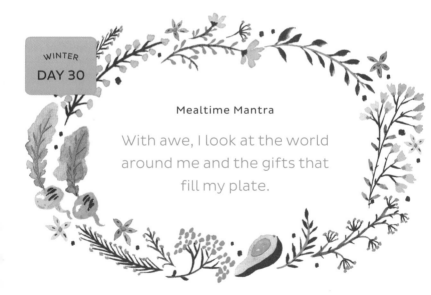

Mealtime Mantra

With awe, I look at the world around me and the gifts that fill my plate.

Kitchen Inspiration

HEALTHY PROTEIN POWDERS

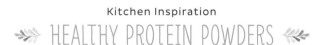

Getting your protein from whole-food sources, like hemp seeds, quinoa, wild salmon, beans, and pastured eggs, is always preferable to processed sources. But when it comes to smoothies and snacks, protein powders are a convenient add-in. When selecting a protein powder, keep a few things in mind. First, quality is your top concern. Look for an organic protein source that's made from whole foods and minimally processed. There are some benefits to whey protein, but I opt for a plant-based protein powder instead, since those are dairy-free and easy to digest. Look for a blend of plant proteins like hemp, rice, and pea, or sprouted rice (skip soy here, as it's often highly processed in powdered form). Depending on your tastes, you may also want to look for protein powder that has a natural sweetener like stevia added, but skip artificial sweeteners like sucralose. You may also find that high-quality protein powders have added benefits like natural digestive enzymes and greens added. They're great to reach for when your fridge is bare and you need some beautifying nutrition in a smoothie.

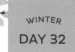
Time for Self-Love

SOAK IN THE WINTER

Taking a bath is one of the most indulgent beauty rituals, but for some of us, some of the time, paradoxically it is perhaps one of the hardest—simply because it requires us to be still and present with our bodies. Soaking in a warm bath is especially restorative during the colder months, when our muscles are sore and tired and the nights are long and dark. Just ten minutes in a bath prepares us for a deep and restful night of beauty sleep. Your skin has a strong power to absorb, so any precious essential oils, salts, or herbs that you use in your bath will work their therapeutic magic both inside and outside of your body. The warmth of the water increases your circulation to give you a digestive and immunity boost, dilates your blood vessels, lowers your blood pressure, and floods your body with warmth. Depending on the temperature of your bath, you may start to sweat, which indicates a boost in your internal detox processes as well. When you leave the water, the subsequent drop in body temperature sends you into a sleep-ready state of calm. Your cortisol drops measurably, and your skin is ready for a massage with natural oils to restore any lost moisture. Drink a glass of room temperature water afterward to rehydrate from the inside as well.

Living Your Best Life

HOW TO MAKE A COLD-FIGHTING ROOM FRESHENER

Help keep your home or office space germ-free this winter with a room-freshening spray that fights bacteria and viruses. In a glass spray bottle, mix ½ cup [240 ml] distilled water with 1 Tbsp rubbing alcohol (used to preserve the formula and disperse the oils), then add about ten drops each of your favorite germ-fighting essential oils, such as tea tree, clove, eucalyptus, juniper, lavender, and/or lemon. Shake well, then spray around your office, bedroom, or anywhere you want to fight germs naturally while freshening your air space—without the harmful chemicals that can be found in synthetic fragrance sprays.

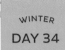
Beauty Food Profile

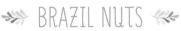

BRAZIL NUTS

Just one incredibly beautifying Brazil nut, so named because it only grows around the Amazon basin, holds your complete daily dose of one of the most important minerals for beauty and anti-aging: selenium. Selenium is anti-inflammatory, protective of the elasticity of our skin, immune- and thyroid-supporting, and defensive against free-radical damage, as well as an important cofactor for the production of the antioxidant glutathione. Brazil nuts are rich in healthy fats that nourish supple skin and strong cell membranes, and they pack in about 1 g of protein per nut. One thing to note is that, while selenium is a powerful beauty mineral, *too much* selenium actually has negative effects for beauty and health. Cap your Brazil nut intake at around four per day.

EAT PRETTY FOOD	BEAUTIFYING COMPOUND	BEAUTY BENEFIT
Brazil nuts	Selenium	Helps maintain skin elasticity

Kitchen Inspiration

ALTERNATIVE CALCIUM SOURCES

Dairy products, even organic versions, contain growth hormones that can throw off your body's own hormonal balance; conventional—meaning non-organic—dairy products are often additionally a source of unwanted antibiotics. Studies linking acne with milk consumption further support that dairy, a common food intolerance, may not be a beauty food at all. The next question is: where can we get calcium if not from dairy? Try sardines, collard greens, bok choy, almonds, figs, chia seeds, amaranth, kale, and white beans for nourishing, frequently forgotten sources of the mineral.

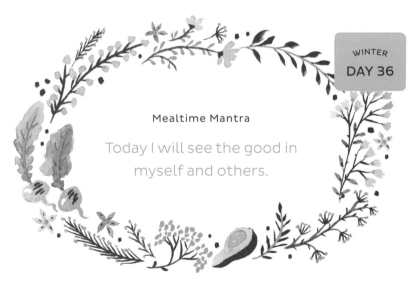

Mealtime Mantra

Today I will see the good in myself and others.

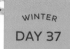
Intention of the Week

EAT MORE CRUCIFEROUS VEGETABLES

Cruciferous vegetables, the family that includes broccoli, cauliflower, and a host of other beauty superfoods, are incredibly powerful tools for healthy aging. Cruciferous vegetables contain phytochemicals called isothiocyanates, which activate Nrf2, a transcription factor that turns on protective genes associated with antioxidant power and lower inflammation. This family of veggies can also detox excess estrogens from the body that can negatively impact mood and weight and increase risk of breast and ovarian cancers. And while we sometimes *think* we eat plenty of our cruciferous favorites, we often come up short. This week, go for extra helpings of Brussels sprouts, kale, arugula, and cauliflower. Seek out bok choy, broccoli rabe, collard greens, kohlrabi, radishes, and horseradish if they haven't landed on your plate in awhile. And know that every bite is brimming with the power to help you age well.

Beauty Science

BLOOD SUGAR AND SKIN AGING

Riding through life on a blood sugar rollercoaster is a bad habit that plagues so many of us, leaving us feeling fuzzy-headed, sapped of energy, and craving sugar and simple carbs, all of which make it harder for us to lose weight, and even put us at risk for diabetes. You should also know that, according to scientific research, mismanaged blood sugar meddles with the healthy aging of your skin. In one study, participants with the highest blood sugar levels were found to show the most signs of skin aging, suggesting the effects of elevated blood sugar over time. One possible cause is glycation, a process by which sugar in your bloodstream attaches to protein molecules, which causes the breakdown of collagen, loss of skin elasticity, wrinkling, and premature signs of aging in the skin. Eating fewer simple carbs and sugars and adding protein and healthy fats to each meal is an important step toward controlling your blood sugar more consistently—and supporting gorgeous, healthy aging!

Eat Pretty Recipe

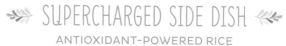

SUPERCHARGED SIDE DISH

ANTIOXIDANT-POWERED RICE

This beautifying rice recipe is adapted from a dish my mother created, which quickly became a favorite healthy comfort food at family gatherings. Its anti-inflammatory, antioxidant, immune-boosting beauty nutrition is as potent as it is delicious. For a festive version of this rice to serve at your holiday table, add ½ cup [50 g] halved fresh cranberries to the pan and cook with the shallots and mushrooms.

SERVES 6

1 tsp coconut oil
2 medium shallots, minced
4 oz [115 g] shiitake mushroom caps, brushed clean and chopped
Pinch of dried marjoram
Pinch of dried tarragon
1½-in [4-cm] knob of fresh ginger, peeled and finely grated

3 cups [555 g] cooked organic short-grain brown rice or 3 cups [345 g] cooked quinoa
2-in [5-cm] knob of fresh turmeric, peeled and finely grated
½ cup [15 g] packed fresh parsley leaves, finely chopped
Unrefined salt and freshly ground black pepper

In a sauté pan or skillet over medium heat, melt the coconut oil. Add the shallots and cook until golden, about 5 minutes. Add the mushrooms, marjoram, tarragon, and ginger and cook, stirring frequently, until the mushrooms are tender and nicely browned. Add the rice and cook, stirring, until heated through. Transfer the mixture to a serving bowl and stir in the turmeric and parsley. Season with salt and pepper. Serve immediately.

Time for Self-Love
STRETCH IT OUT

Sitting all day is not only boring—it's a real downer for your long-term beauty. Sitting for long periods slows down metabolism, circulation, and brain function and negatively impacts our ability to control blood sugar, all of which have damaging effects on the way we look, feel, and age. Since many of us have no choice but to sit for much of our workday, it helps to know a quick series of circulation-boosting stretches to do periodically through-out the day. For an easy regimen, try this sequence: Stand up and reach your arms above you. Bend deeply at the waist and grab your legs, hugging them as closely as you can while you breathe and hold the pose; this will bring blood flow to your head. Slowly straighten, unrolling your spine vertebrae by vertebrae. Put your hands on your waist and extend your right leg in out front of you. Hold this pose for ten seconds. Without touching the ground with your foot, pull in your leg and extend it backward for ten seconds. Then extend it out to the side, holding for ten more seconds. Return your leg to the floor and repeat on the left side. If stretching doesn't feel intensive enough, or for another convenient way to get out of your seat, consider getting a small rebounder (a mini trampoline) for your workspace and spending a few minutes bouncing to rev up both circulation and lymph flow periodically.

Pretty Pairing

❧ QUINOA + GARLIC ❧

Why they're more beautiful together: Sulfur-rich garlic helps the body absorb more of quinoa's powerful beauty minerals: iron and zinc. And together, these beauty superfoods create an antioxidant-packed combo that's also a source of complete protein—a beauty must-have at every meal for building hair, nails, and skin, as well as fighting visible signs of aging.

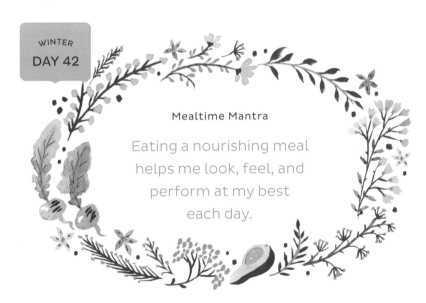

Mealtime Mantra

Eating a nourishing meal
helps me look, feel, and
perform at my best
each day.

Kitchen Inspiration

WINTER SMOOTHIE ESSENTIALS

Winter menus are loaded with meals that are warm and often heavy. When your body craves a cool, light meal or you need nourishment on the go, create a smoothie tailored to the beauty needs of the winter season with these five ingredients: fresh or ground turmeric or ginger, to reduce inflammation and fight colds (try ½ tsp in a serving); raw sauerkraut, to build up immunity-supporting gut bacteria (1 heaping Tbsp in a green smoothie won't change the taste too much, while conferring major benefits); mushroom powder, to support immune function (½ to 1 tsp, depending on the type); and raw cacao powder, for energy and skin hydration (this ingredient does contain caffeine, so start with ½ to 1 tsp, depending on your caffeine tolerance). Adding one or more of these beauty superfoods helps keep you looking and feeling your best through a season that can be filled with pitfalls for our skin and our overall health.

Beauty Food Profile

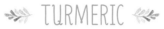

TURMERIC

This bitter root is a source of the strongly antioxidant and anti-inflammatory phytochemical curcumin. The anti-inflammatory powers of curcumin are so great that it's been found to reduce pain even better than several over-the-counter pain relievers. Traditionally, turmeric has been prized for its ability to support metabolism and a healthy weight, heal digestive issues (it may reduce inflammation in the gut) and wounds, and clear up skin issues (it's often used in topical masks for acne). I recommend eating some of this incredibly anti-aging spice every single day, for head-to-toe beauty benefits. Fresh turmeric root has a slightly floral scent that I love in my morning lemon water, and the ground spice works well in stir-fries, curries, and even sprinkled in smoothies and on avocado toast.

EAT PRETTY FOOD	BEAUTIFYING COMPOUND	BEAUTY BENEFIT
Turmeric	Curcumin	Reduces inflammation

Living Your Best Life

HOW TO MAKE YOUR OWN BEAUTIFYING BATH SALTS

I find a beautiful jar of bath salts to be one of the most pampering beauty products you can own (especially if you choose one without synthetic fragrance, color, and potentially toxic preservatives). Fortunately, it's also one of the easiest to make, for yourself and others. Start with a bag of mineral-rich Epsom salts, which are inexpensive and available at the drugstore and online. From there, add smaller quantities of baking soda (for skin-softening), sea salt (for additional minerals), and clays (also mineral-rich and healing). Customize even further with dried flower petals or herbs (lavender is a go-to, but mint and basil are also lovely). You can add your favorite essential oils right into the mixture, or wait and sprinkle them into your bath. A large scoop of these DIY bath salts makes a beautiful, and beautifying, bath.

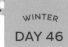
Intention of the Week

AVOID EATING WITHIN TWO HOURS OF BEDTIME

It's common to grab something sweet or crunchy in the evening, while you're reading a book, watching a movie, or out late with friends. But be aware of how often you eat a meal close to bedtime. Eating late saps restorative energy from your body by committing it to digestion, stealing precious hours when your body would normally focus solely on rejuvenation and repair. It's true that eating late once in a while doesn't cause harm, and a small snack before bedtime can actually stabilize blood sugar and help you sleep better if you're hungry, but eating a late meal every night takes a real toll on your beauty sleep. When you give your body adequate time to digest and fast overnight, you awaken ready for an energizing beauty breakfast the next morning. Support optimal rest and repair by not eating within two hours of bedtime this week, and try to continue the practice as often as possible in the future.

Kitchen Inspiration

SIP DIGESTIVE TEA

Stock your kitchen with a tea that supports digestion and you'll support a glowing complexion at the same time. You can readily purchase premade organic ginger teas, which contain phytochemicals that relax stomach muscles and relieve indigestion. Or you can make your own blend by combining fennel seeds, cardamom pods, and dehydrated ginger (either store-bought or homemade from the pulp that remains when you juice a knob of fresh ginger) with a caffeine-free, antioxidant-rich tea like rooibos.

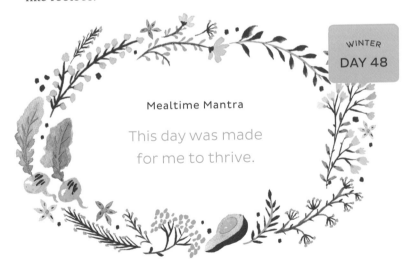

WINTER
DAY 48

Mealtime Mantra

This day was made
for me to thrive.

Time for Self-Love

CONSIDERING A.M. EXERCISE

Ever plan to exercise in the morning, only to find that you can't muster the energy to get out from under the covers? Sometimes there are major benefits to heeding the signals your body is sending—and staying in bed for a little extra beauty sleep! The beauty benefits of sleep are profound, from anti-aging hormone secretion to cell repair, and getting extra zzz's can help restore, recharge, and support a healthy weight in its own way. Of course, don't skip the workout *every* day, but give yourself more restful time when you truly need it—without the guilt.

Eat Pretty Recipe

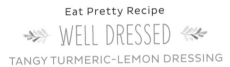

WELL DRESSED

TANGY TURMERIC-LEMON DRESSING

A good dressing transforms the taste of simple foods. A really good dressing transforms their beauty benefits as well! I love the taste of turmeric paired with the sweetness of honey and the lightness of lemon in this dressing. Pour it on your salads, beauty bowls, and stir-fries to up their anti-aging, anti-inflammatory ante.

MAKES ¾ CUP DRESSING

6 Tbsp olive oil
¼ cup [60 ml] fresh lemon juice
2 Tbsp tahini
2 tsp ground turmeric

1 tsp raw honey
Pinch of ground ginger
Pinch of unrefined salt

In a small bowl or jar, whisk or shake together all of the ingredients. Use right away, or cover the bowl or jar tightly and store in the refrigerator for up to 1 week.

Living Your Best Life

HOW TO BREATHE EASIER THIS WINTER

Though it might not seem very glamorous, nasal rinsing is an unquestionable boon to your winter beauty. The defense against and relief from colds and flu that a regular nasal rinse provides is worth a few slightly uncomfortable minutes in front of the mirror as water comes out of your nose. Here's why it works: In the winter, cold, dry air wreaks havoc on our nasal passages, leaving them inflamed and without their healthy moisture and fully functioning cilia that filter harmful bacteria. Nasal rinsing reduces inflammation in dry nasal passages and restores moisture, helping your natural defenses function well once more. My favorite nasal-rinse formula to use during cold season contains naturally virus- and bacteria-fighting essential oils and extracts that work against the itchy, stuffy nose that can be an early sign of a cold. Red nose, avoided.

Beauty Food Profile

TEMPEH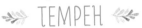

Although there is much debate about the health benefits of soy overall, there are clear beauty benefits to be had from *organic, whole, fermented* soy in the form of organic tempeh, a fermented soybean cake. Tempeh is a major source of protein (about 16 g in a 3-oz/85-g serving), as well as calcium, iron, and vitamin K_2, all made more easily digestible and absorbable by the fermentation process. The whole soybeans in tempeh contain compounds called phytoestrogens, including lignans, that may have a regulative effect on estrogen levels in the body. Studies show that phytoestrogens in soy do not increase, and may even decrease, the risk of breast cancer. Protein from soy has also been found to have an anti-inflammatory effect on the body. To retain the most nutritional value in your tempeh, marinate it to add flavor and then lightly cook it over low heat.

EAT PRETTY FOOD	BEAUTIFYING COMPOUND	BEAUTY BENEFIT
Tempeh	Protein	Building block of beauty

Beauty Science

REST TO RESIST WRINKLES

Research shows that the skin of women who sleep less is more prone to fine lines, less elasticity, and uneven pigmentation. But women who sleep more hours arm themselves with stronger defenses against sun and environmental damage. Since sleep provides free anti-aging (during sleep, your body secretes human growth hormone, or HGH, which increases skin cell production, collagen, and damage repair), aim for seven to nine hours of nightly rest, and take short naps during the day if you're feeling sleep-deprived.

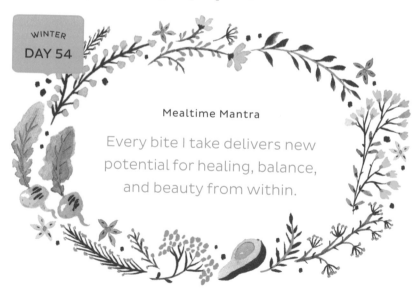

Mealtime Mantra

Every bite I take delivers new
potential for healing, balance,
and beauty from within.

Intention of the Week

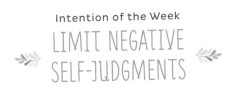

LIMIT NEGATIVE
SELF-JUDGMENTS

How many times have you scolded yourself for eating
something, just a moment or two after swallowing? How
often have you described yourself using ultra-critical
judgments that you would never inflict upon others? This
week, stop yourself whenever you start to say or think
negative statements about your body or your food choices.
If you're going to eat a dish of ice cream, love it. If you're
going to wear a body-conscious dress, own it. The habit of
letting negative thoughts and words populate your day does
more to tear you down than you realize. Making an effort
to change your mindset can reinvent your relationship
with food and open your eyes to your incredible beauty.

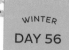

Kitchen Inspiration
BUILD A BETTER PIE CRUST

Classic butter pie crusts are timeless favorites, but contain ingredients that can betray your beauty. This winter, create a crust that is just as delicious but more beauty-friendly with a few simple ingredient swaps. Instead of using white or wheat flour, use nutrient-dense ingredients as the base of your crust. Raw nuts are a go-to for their megadose of beauty nutrients; plus their natural oils help your crust bind together. Gluten-free oats, shredded coconut, or coconut flour help bulk up any crust recipe; I suggest adding those in equal parts to your nuts. Next, incorporate some sticky natural sweetness like dates, raisins, dried figs, or raw honey that will further bring together your dough. Don't forget a little unrefined salt to balance out the sweetness, and any spices or other flavors you wish to add to complement your filling. Use a food processor to pulse all of the ingredients together until they form a sticky dough. Then press into your favorite pie dish for a skin-friendly raw crust that can be filled with fruit or a fancy no-bake filling.

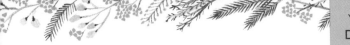

Time for Self-Love

≫ LET GO OF NECK TENSION ≪

Tightness in your neck causes pain above (headaches) and below (sore shoulders and back), as well as poor posture. Actively preventing the buildup of neck tension doesn't have to be complicated; even a one-minute stretch break can loosen clenched muscles and prevent cumulative aches and pains. During your self-care minute, experience the benefits of cat-cow pose: Get down on all fours, with your arms aligned under your shoulders and your legs aligned under your hips. Breathe in through your nose and look up as you arch your back and let your belly sag—like a cow. Feel the stretch through the front of your neck and your stomach muscles? Hold for a moment, then switch to a cat stretch: breathe out through your mouth as you round your back and look downward, stretching the back of your neck and your spine. Alternate through cow and cat stretches several times, ending by sitting back on your heels while folding forward onto the floor—the yogic child's pose. Do this simple stretch daily, and whenever your neck feels tight.

Beauty Science

THE UNEXPECTED BEAUTY BENEFITS OF CHOCOLATE

Here's the best news you'll hear all day: dark chocolate has been scientifically proven to lower levels of the stress hormone cortisol and epinephrine, which, when left unchecked, contribute to wrinkles, skin redness and sensitivity, breakouts, and weight gain. The study that reported these findings used 50 g (or a little less than 2 oz, about half a standard-size bar) of 72 percent dark chocolate (the darker and less processed the better for beauty) and also documented that the participants who consumed dark chocolate reported feeling less stressed during a difficult exercise. Those who ate a placebo that smelled and tasted like dark chocolate but was missing the cocoa flavonols had significantly higher levels of cortisol and epinephrine, showing that the cocoa phytochemicals were the key to increased calm.

Living Your Best Life

HOW TO DETOX YOUR COUNTERTOPS

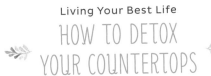

The average store-bought disinfecting soaps, sprays, and other home cleansers are hidden sources of chemicals that can disrupt hormonal balance and your microbiome even as they wipe out countertop germs. To keep germs in check naturally and protect your home environment, make your own cleaning spray or look for a natural brand with botanical germ killers like lavender, oregano, and thyme to disinfect without introducing hormone-disrupting compounds onto surfaces that you, your family, and your foods touch daily.

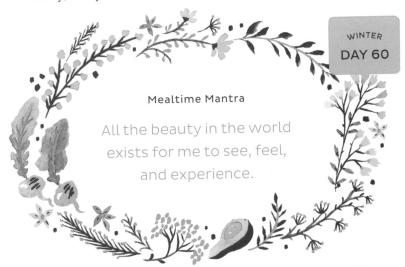

Mealtime Mantra

All the beauty in the world exists for me to see, feel, and experience.

Intention of the Week

FINE-TUNE YOUR FAT INTAKE

Eating fats is essential for supple, well-hydrated skin, healthy hormones, energy, satiety—even maintaining a healthy weight! But the wrong sources of fat—like fried foods cooked in heated oils, processed or bleached cooking oils, and foods that contain an overabundance of omega-6 fats—will burden you with large quantities of free radicals and contributors to inflammation and hormonal imbalance. This week's challenge comes in two parts: one, add more healthy fats to your diet (think avocado, coconut oil, hemp seeds, raw nuts, wild salmon, and flaxseeds), and two, reduce the amount of unhealthy fats you consume (skip the fries, roasted nuts, processed snacks, premade salad dressings, and tempura anything—even if it's veggies). It's hard to control the type of fats you're eating in most restaurants, so, if you have plans to dine out, expect that you won't be able to eliminate unhealthy fats 100 percent. Use the week as an exercise in awareness of the places where you can go out of your way to nourish your beauty with delicious, healthy fat sources.

Beauty Food Profile

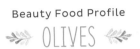 OLIVES

Olives are about 88 percent fat (the healthy kind), making them an excellent beauty food for the skin. The fats in olives include vitamin E, a strong antioxidant that supports healthy levels of anti-aging glutathione in the body; oleic acid, a monounsaturated fat that also makes olive oil a superfood; and alpha-linolenic acid, used to make omega-3 fats in the body. In concert, these fats create a strong nutritional boost that strengthens cell membranes, regulates oil production, and reduces allergies and inflammation. In fact, olives contain an anti-inflammatory compound called oleocanthal, also found in olive oil, that has been shown to rival the anti-inflammatory properties of over-the-counter drugs. Snack on a few of these beautifying, and satisfying, fruits when you're hungry in between meals.

EAT PRETTY FOOD	BEAUTIFYING COMPOUND	BEAUTY BENEFIT
Olives	Vitamin E	Supports glutathione production in the body

Eat Pretty Recipe

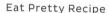# SWEET A.M. PROTEIN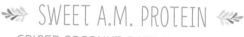

SPICED COCONUT-DATE AMARANTH

All beauty breakfasts call for protein and healthy fats, and in winter, they call for an extra dash of warmth. This naturally sweet dish hits every spot, with 10 grams of protein per serving and skin-nourishing coconut in a comforting hot cereal. If you're short on time in the morning, make a batch at the beginning of the week and reheat it, serving by serving, with a little extra coconut milk.

SERVES 4

3 cups [720 ml] water
⅓ cup [50 g] chopped dates
¼ tsp unrefined salt
1½ tsp ground cinnamon
½ tsp ground cardamom

1 cup [200 g] amaranth
2 Tbsp plus 2 tsp shelled
  hemp seeds
½ cup [120 ml] coconut milk
4 tsp coconut butter (optional)

In a medium saucepan, combine the water, dates, and salt and bring to a boil. Add the cinnamon, cardamom, and amaranth, reduce the heat, and simmer until the cereal thickens, about 20 minutes. Remove from the heat and divide into four servings. Top each serving with 2 tsp hemp seeds, 2 Tbsp coconut milk, and 1 tsp coconut butter and serve.

Time for Self-Love

FIND BARE-FACED BEAUTY

How often do you let your face go naked? Our skin benefits from periodic stretches of time to breathe and renew—hence the importance of taking off your makeup at night. This winter, try to set aside some time at regular intervals to let your skin breathe, makeup free. Cleanse your face, apply your moisturizer (to combat the drying effects of indoor heated air), then cozy up with a favorite at-home activity as your skin basks in its natural state. You'll benefit physically from the makeup free moments (your skin absorbs 60 percent of the ingredients you apply to it, so it could use a break now and then) and also emotionally, since seeing—and loving—your face without makeup can help you adore the skin you're in. And when you choose to make up your face again, the effect will be all the more dramatic and special.

Kitchen Inspiration

REACH FOR RAW NUTS

Grabbing a package of roasted nuts feels like a healthy choice, but it's not the best bet for your skin. When delicate nut oils are heated to high temps during the roasting process, or left to hang out on shelves for weeks after roasting, they can go rancid and produce additional aging free radicals in your body when you eat them. Get in the habit of buying raw nuts and seeds, and storing them in the freezer to protect their oils. You'll fill up on beautifying fats in their highest form.

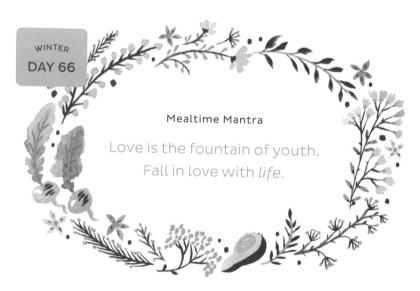

Mealtime Mantra

Love is the fountain of youth.
Fall in love with *life*.

Time for Self-Love

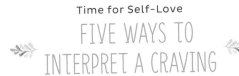

FIVE WAYS TO INTERPRET A CRAVING

Can you tell me what you ate last weekend? How about yesterday? In the moment, food—especially foods we crave—can be all-consuming, but a few days or even a few moments later, we've forgotten why we needed it so badly. Next time you feel a craving or impulse to grab something that you know won't make you feel your best later, pause. Ask yourself, is your craving actually a sign of:

1. Stress?
2. Hunger for real nutrients—especially lack of protein and healthy fats?
3. Your body's need for energy because of a blood sugar spike and crash?
4. A need for self-love, or something to make you feel cared for?
5. Imbalance somewhere else in your life?

If you realize yes, you are actually just feeling stressed, or overworked, or in need of a little pampering, take a moment to schedule in what it is you *really* need. And when you do splurge or indulge in a craving, make it something you'll enjoy the memory of even a week later.

Living Your Best Life

HOW TO KEEP SKIN HYDRATED THIS SEASON

Indoor air, hot water, alcohol, sugar, air travel, and caffeine are some of the biggest culprits behind dry skin. It's no wonder that this season, when you're hanging out indoors, taking hot showers to warm up, celebrating with cocktails and cookies, traveling long distances to see family, and sipping lattes to stay energized, you start to see major signs of skin dryness! Skip parched skin by cutting back on the Beauty Betrayers (like alcohol, caffeine, sugar, and processed foods), setting up a humidifier in your workspace or bedroom (or both), eating plenty of healthy fats, and regularly applying a natural moisturizer with plant-based oils or butters. Keep drinking water as well—in the form of herbal teas and warm lemon water as well as room temperature water—and you'll see suppler skin this season.

Intention of the Week
CULTIVATE HEALTHY
BEAUTY SLEEP HABITS

No matter what, at least one-third of my day, every day, is *completely* devoted to beauty. Of course, I'm not awake during that time. My sleep hours—and yours—are a built-in beauty reset meant to be used to its fullest every night. That means getting to bed before I get that nightly surge of cortisol that makes it harder to fall asleep. It also means sipping tea or taking a bath to get into rest mode, not eating right before bedtime to allow my body to digest food completely and create time for true rest, and shutting off my computer and smartphone as early as I can before bedtime (this is hard, but I *try*). This week, I challenge you to do the same. Create a nightly pattern that you can practice often to squeeze every ounce of anti-aging power out of your nightly beauty reset. Sleep is extra important during the winter season, so listen to nature and get to bed early!

Kitchen Inspiration

DRINK HOT WATER

How often do you reach for plain, hot water? Rarely, if ever, I'm going to guess. But you're missing out on a powerful detox drink! Sipping hot water is a time-honored way of supporting detox, digestion, and beauty by increasing circulation, encouraging elimination, and stimulating the flow of waste-removing lymph throughout the body. This winter, when circulation and lymph flow are often at their slowest, sip hot water instead of cold throughout the day (add a squeeze of lemon or a pinch of ground ginger if you want a hint of flavor).

Beauty Science
⟫ CALM DOWN TO WAKE UP ⟪

Meditation, gentle yoga practice, and body-scanning exercises (such as consciously relaxing your muscles, starting with the toes and moving upward throughout the body) significantly increase energy and well-being and reduce stress and depression, according to scientific study. One of the most important components of these practices is your breath, since deep, slow breathing increases your oxygen intake for a boost in energy and circulation of well-oxygenated blood. Next time you need to focus deeply, or perform at the top of your game, slow down first.

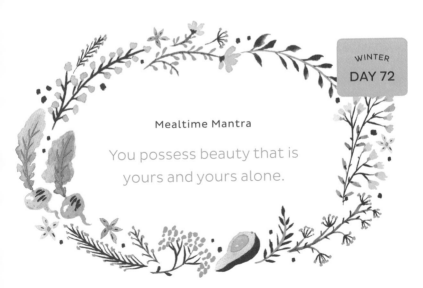

Mealtime Mantra

You possess beauty that is
yours and yours alone.

Living Your Best Life

HOW TO ENJOY A WINTER RETREAT

Wintertime is packed with spirited celebrations, but it's also the season to do a bit of resting and resetting for the health of your beauty and body. Carve out an evening, a day, or a weekend at home or in a peaceful setting during which you can retreat from the world and honor your body's season of rest. Rather than curling up on the couch in front of the television, retreating means actively taking care of your needs and using your time away to accomplish true mind-body replenishment. Sleep as much as you need, eat nourishing meals, meditate and enjoy creative activities like reading or painting, spend time in nature, and take care of your body with rituals like dry brushing, steaming, soaking, and applying natural skincare products. Use your reset time to set intentions for the rest of the winter season, so that you feel ready to embrace spring when it arrives.

Beauty Food Profile

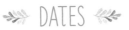

DATES

A beauty-friendly sweet treat, dates offer fruit sugar with additional benefits, as long as you eat them in moderation. Dates are so concentrated in their levels of fructose and sucrose that just a few of them provide ample sugar when added to a dessert recipe. Additionally, they offer fiber, which helps detoxify the body and stabilize blood sugar, and small amounts of B vitamins, calcium, potassium, and iron. Although there are hundreds of varieties of dates, each with varying nutritional benefits, overall they have been shown to offer antioxidant as well as anti-tumor potential in studies. Pair a few dates with a handful of almonds for a sweet and energizing snack on the go.

EAT PRETTY FOOD	BEAUTIFYING COMPOUND	BEAUTY BENEFIT
Dates	Fiber	Aids in detox

Intention of the Week

PERFORM A POST-BATHING SKIN-CARE RITUAL

Dry skin, a lackluster complexion, dark circles, and congestion in your body are signs that you need a boost in circulation of both lymph and blood this winter. This week, after every shower or bath, take ten minutes to perform a calming, two-part self-care ritual that will speed up circulation, support immunity and hormone balance, and restore glow to your winter-weary skin. You'll need a dry brush (an inexpensive tool that you can find at a drugstore or online) and an organic body oil free of synthetic fragrance. This can be as simple as plain coconut, almond, or sesame oil. After your bath or shower, use your dry brush to gently yet firmly brush your skin, from your hands and feet in toward your heart (see the instructions on page 51). Follow with a five-minute self-massage (called *abhyanga* in the Ayurvedic tradition) in the same direction, with your body oil. Finish by massaging your stomach clockwise with oil. If you're performing this self-care ritual at night, wrap yourself in a robe or cozy pajamas and let the oil fully soak into your skin while you sleep.

Kitchen Inspiration

SOAKING NUTS AND SEEDS

There are two reasons that you may want to soak your nuts and seeds before eating them: to soften them to make a recipe like nut milk, and to reduce their content of natural compounds called enzyme inhibitors, thereby making them more easily digestible. It's not necessary to soak all of your nuts and seeds all the time, but when you do have extra time, it can be a beneficial step in maximizing your beauty nutrition. Put the raw nuts in a bowl, add filtered water to cover, and let them soak several hours or overnight, then rinse well. Afterward, you can use a dehydrator or a low temperature oven to dry the nuts back to crispness, or use them as-is in your recipes.

Time for Self-Love

OWN YOUR POWER

Adopt the mindset that right now, in this very moment, you are full of healing potential. At times our bodies, and our beauty, betray us. We stumble, look the worse for wear, stay in bed and hide under the covers, or are forced to rest and recover. When these moments arrive for you, remember your body's inherent strength and healing capacity instead of feeling frustrated or disheartened. Your body works hard to heal, repair, and thrive. It's your job to honor it with nutrition and lifestyle choices that encourage its beauty and strength.

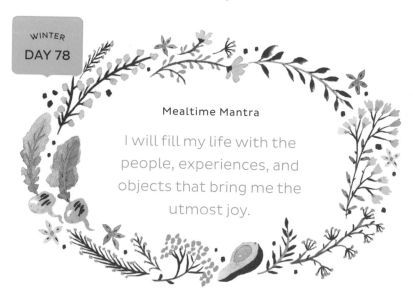

Mealtime Mantra

I will fill my life with the people, experiences, and objects that bring me the utmost joy.

Beauty Science

IN YOUR GENES

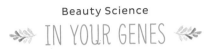

Among the many genes you carry, some specific ones are tied to protein synthesis, to collagen and antioxidant production, to hydration, to inflammation, and to longevity. The foods you eat and the way you care for your body day to day determine whether these genes will be activated, or shut down. Scientific study continues in this exciting area, to determine which foods and habits connect to genes associated with beauty and healthy aging. For example, research already suggests that foods like turmeric, green tea, blueberries, cocoa, pomegranate, cinnamon, and garlic are not just incredibly beautifying because of their antioxidant levels; their phytochemicals also have the power to turn off the transcription factor, known as NF-KB, that activates pro-aging genes, helping you age more beautifully at the genetic level.

Eat Pretty Recipe

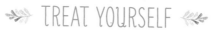

TREAT YOURSELF

SALTED SUPERFOOD CHOCOLATE BARK

It's not just a rumor: chocolate can most definitely be a beauty food! This rich chocolate bark supports skin with a concentrated dose of antioxidants, plus omega-3s and beauty minerals like magnesium and zinc. Make it as decadent as you wish with your choice of raw nuts, seeds, and ground spices, which only add to the beauty benefits.

MAKES A 12-BY-12-IN [30-BY-30-CM] BARK

¾ cup [165 g] coconut butter
½ cup [110 g] coconut oil
⅓ cup [37 g] raw cacao powder or cocoa powder
2 Tbsp maple syrup

5 to 6 drops liquid stevia
Unrefined salt (fine and coarse, for sprinkling)
¼ to ⅓ cup [30 to 40 g] raw walnuts, roughly chopped

In a double boiler, melt the coconut butter and coconut oil. You can achieve this without a double boiler by partially submerging a heat-proof bowl in a pan full of hot water on your stovetop, stirring until the coconut butter and oil are fully melted. Remove from the heat and stir in the raw cacao, maple syrup, stevia, and a pinch of fine salt. On a parchment-lined baking sheet, spread the melted mixture to desired thickness and top with a sprinkling of coarse salt, walnuts, and any other desired add-ins. Be sure to press the nuts into the mixture. Transfer to the freezer for 30 minutes or until solid. Break apart into chunks and serve straight from the freezer.

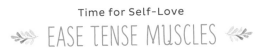

Time for Self-Love

EASE TENSE MUSCLES

Sore muscles bother us all at times, whether it's after a workout, during a stressful day at work, or in the middle of a cold winter when we tense them more because of the cold temperatures. Explore new ways to counter minor aches and pains naturally during this season of cold, using spices, mineral-rich salts, and essential oils as a first line of defense. Turmeric often produces powerful relief for muscle aches, thanks to its strong anti-inflammatory properties. Try adding more of the fresh spice to your meals and making a tonic of fresh, grated turmeric and warm water with a little raw honey. For more pronounced stiffness or soreness, a soak in a hot bath containing magnesium-rich Epsom salts can release tension immediately. And finally, look for muscle-relaxing massage oils (my favorites come in roll-on applicators to get right into your sore spots) that contain essential oils like birch and lavender, known to relieve muscle tension. Use them for self-massage wherever you feel a nagging ache.

Intention of the Week

STABILIZE YOUR BLOOD SUGAR

When was the last time you felt "hangry," that feeling of frustration and even anger that you get when you're hungry? Or experienced an energy slump at three p.m.? Or had uncontrollable cravings? In those moments, you played victim to out-of-balance blood sugar. Eating to support steady blood sugar, thereby minimizing its highs and lows, has a profound impact on your skin, weight, energy, and moods. Managing blood sugar takes some practice, since it's not something that many of us are typically conscious of, but it's worth the effort! This week, start paying attention to your blood sugar by following these concepts: Make sure all of your meals contain vegetables along with protein and healthy fats (which are slower burning foods with a lower glycemic load, a measure of the body's blood sugar response) to steady your blood sugar and keep you full. Don't skip meals. If you're facing an extended period of time between meals that can't be avoided, eat a protein-rich snack. Choose whole foods, which tend to have a lower glycemic load, and sparingly eat foods with a high glycemic load like processed snacks, sweets, simple carbs, alcohol, and coffee. Eat a protein-rich breakfast soon after waking to start off the day with energy. This new way of thinking about your body's response to food can truly transform the way you look and feel.

Pretty Pairing

ORGANIC KALE + AVOCADO

Why they're more beautiful together: Top your kale salad with chunks of creamy avocado to help your body absorb more of the skin-beautifying carotenoids found in this powerful leafy green. When eaten together, the healthy fats in avocado leave you feeling satiated and allow more of the carotenoids found in kale to be used by your body, where they assist with actions like repairing skin cells, balancing oil production in the skin, and defending against UV damage.

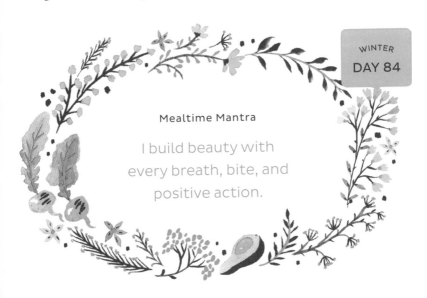

Mealtime Mantra

I build beauty with every breath, bite, and positive action.

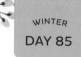
Living Your Best Life

HOW TO FIND A BEAUTIFUL SLEEPING POSITION

Many beauty experts recommend sleeping on your back to keep the weight of your head (about 8 lb/3.6 kg) from putting sustained pressure on your delicate facial skin, causing wrinkles in the long run. If you're comfortable sleeping in that position, more power to you! But what about those who just can't seem to sleep lying face up? All things considered, sleeping *well* each night is much more important for beauty than sleeping on your back. Try getting comfy by lying on your side with a pillow that keeps your neck in a neutral position (not raised or lowered), then place a small pillow between your knees to keep your lower spine neutral, and hug a firm pillow that allows you to comfortably rest your upper arms. Sleeping with so many pillows may sound complicated, but cradling your body in plush feels like sleeping on clouds. Try it and you could get better beauty sleep tonight!

Beauty Food Profile

GREEN TEA

This beauty brew offers a strong concentration of anti-oxidants that have been studied for their diverse anti-aging, health-supporting properties. When it comes to beauty, you want to be a green tea drinker for the wrinkle-reducing, sun-protective benefits in each cup. Phyto-chemicals in green tea called catechins (the best-known being EGCG) have the potential to block the wrinkle-forming process in the body, reverse damage caused by sun exposure, and even prevent DNA damage and the formation of skin cancer. All the while, the antioxidants in green tea have shown an ability to revive dying skin cells and defend against free-radical damage from daily stress and outside sources like pollution, slowing down the aging process overall.

EAT PRETTY FOOD	BEAUTIFYING COMPOUND	BEAUTY BENEFIT
Green tea	EGCG	Blocks a wrinkle-forming process in the body

Kitchen Inspiration

KITCHEN FLEXIBILITY

Let's be honest, not everyone finds joy in cooking meals from scratch day after day. When you're tired, or feeling uninspired, honor the rest you need. Keep what brings you joy and let everything else go. Of course, it's often in our depleted moments that we need beauty nutrition the most. So, what are the ways that you can heed your need for rest while still getting beautifying nutrition? Know at least a few healthy takeout spots or cafés where you can get your beauty foods to go. Buy prechopped veggies so the prep work is done for you. Consider a healthy meal-delivery or meal-planning service for busy times. Sometimes, perfect really is the enemy of the good, and getting healthy beauty fuel in your body (and time out to rest and recharge) matters more than whether or not you cooked it yourself.

Intention of the Week

REPURPOSE LEFTOVERS TO MAKE BEAUTIFYING MEALS

Utilizing leftovers is so satisfyingly economical; you cook once and eat two or even three times, spending less time in the kitchen and ensuring that no beauty nutrient goes to waste. This week, get creative with your leftovers. Eat dinner leftovers for breakfast (protein-rich dinners like wild salmon or quinoa make ideal energizers first thing in the morning), or add them to a few handfuls of fresh greens for lunch. Transform them by drizzling them with a superfood dressing, or slather them with hummus and roll them into a collard wrap. Broadening your repertoire of ways to use leftovers means that beautifying nutritional value goes further, and you'll have less work to do to nourish your skin and body each day.

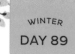

Beauty Science

MOOD-BOOSTING MOUTHFULS

Research shows that a healthy gut does more than support glowing skin and immunity: it actually makes us happier. No surprise, since 50 percent of your dopamine and 95 percent of your serotonin, both happiness neurotransmitters, are produced there. One recent study actually found that after four weeks of a daily probiotic supplement (which supports a healthy gut), participants reported less focus on negative thoughts and experiences. To avoid the dip in mood that often accompanies dreary winter days, fit in a serving of probiotic-rich fermented foods daily.

Time for Self-Love

USE YOUR IMAGINATION

As a child, you probably spent hours visiting far-off places inside your head. As we enter adulthood, reality takes over and we often lose that imagination skill. But being able to flip on your imagination to take you away from an anxiety-filled day is a very important, very beautifying skill for adults. Using your imagination to visualize yourself in a peaceful moment or traveling to an exotic locale elicits some of the same stress-busting effects as deep breathing and meditation. Next time you encounter a stressful feedback loop repeating in your head, let your mind drift . . . imagine yourself in your happy place, exploring a beautiful deserted beach, or reliving a joyful moment, and you'll stop your brain's panic alarm in its tracks.

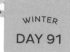
Kitchen Inspiration
SPROUT YOUR WAY TO SPRING

Winter is the season to fortify your body with warm, cooked, nutrient-dense foods (don't you feel cozy just thinking about it?), but it's natural to crave a dose of spring and its fresh, light, crunchy greens while the temps are still frigid. One of my favorite ways to get a sneak preview of spring is to sprout some edible seeds or beans and add them as a crunchy, light, beautifying component to meals. Sprouts are bursting with energy and nutrition for your body and skin; they contain high concentrations of enzymes (absent in cooked food) that help break down food and assimilate nutrients. One of the best sprout varieties for anti-aging, due to its detoxifying and antioxidant-rich sulforaphane, is broccoli sprouts. To experience the satisfaction and major nutrition of sprouting on your own, you can sprout in a jar with a mesh or cheesecloth top, purchase one of any number of sprouting systems, or invest in a simple sprout bag (my favorite method). Once you have your seeds in the bag, it only requires a dip in water twice daily to produce sprouts in three or four days, for most varieties. Give it a try for a low-effort, high-reward way to grow your own beauty food.

HERE'S WHERE WE LEAVE YOU, WINTER. FINALLY, SPRING!

As you come to the end of over ninety entries that spotlight winter beauty practices, do you feel replenished and ready to welcome the rebirth of spring? The cycle begins again in nature, in your body, and in your beauty. Hold onto the moments you've carved out for rest, rejuvenation, nutrition, and self-love, as those are cornerstones of your beautiful life at all times. Continue to surround yourself with the people who support you in maintaining the habits that make you feel good. And get excited about the new year of beauty—foods, recipes, celebrations— you're about to begin. As you move forward, remember to eat the foods and repeat the habits you found to be the most beloved and beautifying, reread your favorite pages of inspiration, and create your own unique practices that support beauty and health, committing once more to do one thing that makes you glow every day in the year ahead. To begin a new season of beautifying inspiration, flip to the start of the Spring chapter on page 21.

ACKNOWLEDGMENTS

When I look through the pages of this book, I can't help but think first of the immense gratitude I feel toward the family and friends who lovingly cared for my little boy while I logged hours in my office researching, writing, and editing. There would be no book without your support. Thank you for making it possible for me to pursue my passion without overwhelming mom guilt!

Immeasurable thanks go to the most talented, humble, and all-around-loveliest editor I have ever worked with, Elizabeth Yarborough. Thank you for your confidence in me and my words, your spot-on insights and edits, and your friendship.

An important thank-you goes to Clare Pelino for joining me on this journey and serving as my sage guide through the publishing world.

To the Chronicle Books team and illustrator Vikki Chu, thank you for devoting your time and talent to building and sharing the books in the *Eat Pretty* collection. Each season, your publications thrill me and remind me why I love books. I'm so grateful to be one of your authors.

To the readers and clients around the globe who have been so passionately sharing, supporting, and living *Eat Pretty*, this book is for you. I'm in awe of your personal transformations and the beauty you possess, inside and out. May you find inspiration and a guiding voice in these pages, plus even more ways to fill your life with beauty.

To my dear parents, thank you for the priceless gifts you've given me, including the confidence and desire to trust and honor my own unique body, mind, and instincts. Thank you, and thank you to my parents-in-law, for your tireless love and support.

And to Rob, your love truly makes it all possible for me. I dream, create, and work toward new goals the way I do because I share my life with you.

REFERENCED STUDIES

Spring

p. 34, regarding chemical detox: "Reducing phthalate, paraben, and phenol exposure from personal care products in adolescent girls: Findings from the HERMOSA Intervention study," *Environmental Health Perspectives*, March 2016.

p. 43, regarding healthy eating at home: "Emotional reinforcement as a protective factor for healthy eating in home settings," *The American Journal of Clinical Nutrition*, May 2011.

p. 49, regarding the source of happiness: "A functional genomic perspective on human well-being," *Proceedings of the National Academy of Sciences*, July 2013.

p. 52, regarding edible flowers: "Phenolic compounds and antioxidant capacities of 10 common edible flowers from China," *Journal of Food Science*, March 2014.

p. 57, regarding crushed garlic: "Recipe for healthy garlic: crush before cooking," *Science Daily*, February 2007.

p. 60, regarding the benefits of journaling: "Emotional and physical health benefits of expressive writing," *Advances in Psychiatric Treatment*, August 2005.

p. 73, regarding a boost in keratin production: "Nutrient supplementation influence on keratinocytes metabolism: an in vitro study," *Surgical and Cosmetic Dermatology*, May 2012.

p. 95, regarding walking and mental well-being: "Physical activity and mental well-being in a cohort aged 60-64 years," *The American Journal of Preventive Medicine*, August 2015.

p. 97, regarding food cravings: "Pilot randomized trial demonstrating reversal of obesity-related abnormalities in reward system responsivity to food cues with a behavioral intervention," *Nutrition & Diabetes*, September 2014.

p. 110, regarding roses: "Effect of rose essential oil inhalation on stress-induced skin barrier disruption in rats and humans," *Chemical Senses*, October 2011. AND "Effect of olfactory stimulation by fresh rose flowers on autonomic nervous system activity," *The Journal of Alternative and Complementary Medicine*, July 2014.

p. 118, regarding black rice and anthocyanins: "Black rice rivals pricey blueberries as source of healthful antioxidants," *Science Daily*, August 2010.

p. 120, regarding skin aging and pH: "The effect of probiotics on immune regulation, acne, and photoaging," *International Journal of Women's Dermatology*, June 2015.

p. 127, regarding urine pesticide levels after eating organic: "Reduction in urinary organophosphate pesticide metabolites in adults after a week-long organic diet," *Environmental Research*, July 2014.

p. 130, regarding stress and digestion: "Exposure to a social stressor alters the structure of the intestinal microbiota: Implications for stressor-induced immunomodulation," *Brain, Behavior, and Immunity*, March 2011.

p. 137, regarding beets and cycling performance: "Dietary nitrate supplementation reduces the O_2 cost of low-intensity exercise and enhances tolerance to high-intensity exercise in humans," *Journal of Applied Physiology*, October 2009.

p. 150, regarding sun-protective foods: "Lycopene-rich products and dietary photoprotection," *Photochemical & Photobiological Sciences*, February 2006. AND "Dietary tomato paste protects against ultraviolet light-induced erythema in humans," *Journal of Nutrition*, May 2001. AND "Protective effect against sunburn of combined systemic ascorbic acid (vitamin C) and d-alpha-tocopherol (vitamin E)," *Journal of the American Academy of Dermatology*, January 1998. AND "Dietary fish-oil supplementation in humans reduces UVB-erythemal sensitivity but increases epidermal lipid peroxidation," *Journal of Investigative Dermatology*, August 1994.

p. 175, regarding leafy greens and digestive health: "YihQ is a sulfoqui-novosidase that cleaves sulfoquinovosyl diaglyceride sulfolipids," *Nature Chemical Biology*, February 2016.

p. 181, regarding incidence of eczema in dishwasher households: "Allergy in children in hand versus machine dishwashing," *Pediatrics*, March 2015.

Autumn

p. 197, regarding stress and beneficial bacteria: "Exposure to a social stressor alters the structure of the intestinal microbiota: Implications for stressor-induced immunomodulation," *Brain, Behavior, and Immunity*, March 2011.

p. 206, regarding multitasking: "Cognitive control in media multitask-ers," *Proceedings of the National Academy of Sciences*, August 2009.

p. 217, regarding napping and cortisol levels: "Benefits of napping and an extended duration of recovery sleep on alertness and immune cells after acute sleep restriction," *Brain, Behavior, and Immunity*, January 2011.

p. 218, regarding probiotics and stress reduction: "Consumption of fermented milk product with probiotic modulates brain activity," *Gastroenterology*, June 2013.

p. 227, regarding blood levels of carotenoids and optimism: "Associa-tion between optimism and serum antioxidants in the midlife in the United States study," *Psychosomatic Medicine*, January 2013.

p. 232, regarding relaxed breathing and glycemic response: "Relaxation breathing improves human glycemic response," *The Journal of Alterna-tive and Complementary Medicine*, July 2013.

p. 234, regarding awe and lowered inflammatory markers: "Positive affect markers of inflammation: Discrete positive emotions predict lower levels of inflammatory cytokines," *Emotion*, January 2015.

p. 238, regarding yoga practice and lowered oxidative stress and adren-aline: "Regular yoga practice improves antioxidant status, immune function, and stress hormone release in young healthy people: a randomized, double-blind, controlled pilot study," *The Journal of Alternative and Complementary Medicine*, July 2015.

p. 242, regarding diet and skin wrinkling: "Skin wrinkling: can food make a difference?" *Journal of the American College of Nutrition*, February 2001.

p. 247, regarding milk consumption and acne: "Role of insulin, insulin-like growth factor-1, hyperglycaemic food and milk consumption in the pathogenesis of acne vulgaris," *Experimental Dermatology*, October 2009.

p. 257, regarding the health benefits of giving a massage: "The benefits of giving a massage on the mental state of massage therapists: a randomized, controlled study," *The Journal of Alternative and Complementary Medicine*, November 2012.

Winter

p. 279, regarding sleep duration and likelihood of catching a cold virus: "Behaviorally assessed sleep and susceptibility to the common cold," *Sleep*, September 2015.

p. 300, regarding phytochemicals in cruciferous vegetables: "Natural products for cancer prevention associated with Nrf2-ARE pathway," *Food Science and Human Wellness*, March 2013.

p. 314, regarding the skin of women who sleep less: "Sleep deprivation linked to aging skin, study suggests," *Science Daily*, July 2013.

p. 318, regarding stress levels after dark chocolate consumption: "Dark chocolate intake buffers stress reactivity in humans," *Journal of the American College of Cardiology*, June 2014.

p. 344, regarding probiotics effect on mood: "A randomized controlled trial to test the effect of multispecies probiotics on cognitive reactivity to sad mood," *Brain, Behavior, and Immunity*, August 2015.

INDEX